The Dance Goes On

THE DANCE GOES ON

ROBERTA BANDY

Rob loved to dance in spite of his severe disabilities. Here's how he brought us joy and taught us about life, love, and God.

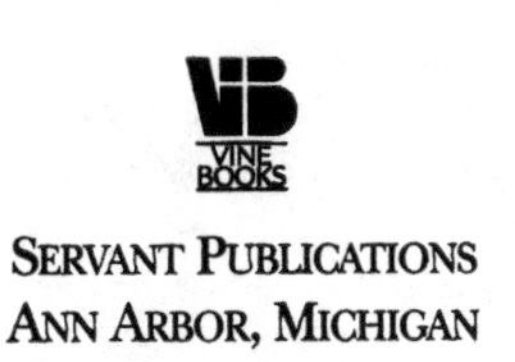

SERVANT PUBLICATIONS
ANN ARBOR, MICHIGAN

Vine Books is an imprint of Servant Publications especially designed to serve evangelical Christians.

Servant Publications—Mission Statement
We are dedicated to publishing books that spread the gospel of Jesus Christ, help Christians to live in accordance with that gospel, promote renewal in the church, and bear witness to Christian unity.

Published in association with Yates and Yates, LLP, Attorneys and Counselors, Orange, California.

Servant Publications
P.O. Box 8617
Ann Arbor, MI 48107
www.servantpub.com

Cover design: Noah Pudgil Design

03 04 05 06 10 9 8 7 6 5 4 3 2 1

Printed in the United States of America
ISBN 1-56955-388-2

Library of Congress Cataloging-in-Publication Data

Bandy, Roberta.
The dance goes on / Roberta Bandy.
p. cm.
ISBN 1-56955-388-2
1. Parents of chronically ill children–Religious life. 2. Chronic diseases in children–Religious aspects–Christianity. I. Title.
BV4596.P33B36 2003
248.8'64'092–dc21

2003012381

Thou mastering me
God! Giver of breath and bread
World's strand, sway of the sea;
Lord of living and dead,
Thou hast bound bones and veins in me, fastened me flesh,
And after it almost unmade, what with dread,
Thy doing: and dost thou touch me afresh?
Over again I feel thy finger and find thee.

From *The Wreck of the Deutschland*
By Gerard Manley Hopkins

Foreword

by Christopher de Vinck

Recently, I was told a wonderful story that took place in the New York City subway system. An old, homeless woman was sprawled out on three seats of a subway car. She was unkempt, nearly toothless, and someone clearly to avoid.

As the train stopped at the next station, a young, confident businessman dressed in a pressed three-piece suit stepped into the subway. When the doors closed, the man held on to a pole to stabilize himself. Suddenly, the old woman looked up and asked the man, "Mister, do you have somethin' to eat?" The man looked down at the disheveled woman and said, "No. I'm sorry."

"Do you got a nickel?" the woman asked.

The man rummaged through his pocket and answered, "No. I don't have any spare change."

The woman then looked up at the man, squinted, and asked, "Well, do you dance?"

I thought about this little story as I finished reading about Rob Bandy. Throughout this book, Rob's mother asks that same question of us all: "Do you dance?"

In the time we give birth to our children, we project all that we believe about life and comfort and stability, and we place these notions into our arms as our new son or daughter is carried home. But what happens when that life, comfort, and stability is threatened each day?

This book is the story of a child born with what doctors

called severe physical impairments, and this is a book about how the boy's mother learns over the twenty-nine years of her son's life that these were not impairments, but distractions to what is central to all human existence: love.

According to Roberta, her son loved the Muppets and the smell of flowers. He laughed easily. She remembers the day her husband and Rob were out on a lake together in a small boat, how Rob affected the lives of his brothers and sisters, and how grand it all was when Rob discovered that he loved to dance.

This is a book about struggle. It is not a book about disabilities—it is about us all. Roberta asks in this spiritually practical book, *Where does hope come from? How,* she asks, *can I get the world to see my son as I see him?* For her it was at the moment when she said to herself, "Thy will be done." Like Roberta, my mother gave birth to my brother Oliver at the end of World War II: blind, disabled, intellectually void Oliver, yet she, too, discovered the same answers Roberta discovered. As my mother stood in the cathedral in Brussels with her sick, hopeless child, she whispered in the shadows of the great church, "Thy will be done," and then my mother spent the next thirty-two years dancing with my brother Oliver, and teaching me and my brothers and sisters to do the same.

This book is not about miracles, or about ways to solve our problems. It is a book that says we all have problems, and how we tend to those problems defines who we are.

Rob's mother clearly states that the flaws she saw in her son were no greater than our own flaws. So what does Roberta offer us here? She says that if we all learn to love the Muppets, and the smell of flowers, if we all learn to laugh easily and to dance, even in the face of our sorrow, we will discover, or rediscover, a purity of heart in ourselves, and it is in that purity of heart where we discover a fine day, or solace, or God.

The next pages will, in Roberta's own words, offer those who have the courage to turn each page "reflections and comfort in the truth of sorrow."

Roberta asks, in the presence of her suffering, in the presence of all of our suffering, "Do you dance?" How we answer that question, as is chronicled in these pages, makes all the difference in the world.

~ ONE ~

Who gave man his mouth? Who makes him deaf or mute? Who gives him sight or makes him blind? Is it not I, the Lord?

EXODUS 4:11

Before I formed you in the womb I knew you, before you were born I set you apart.

JEREMIAH 1:5

His name was Rob. He was our firstborn. His life changed the course of ours and, with God's direction, formed us into the people we have become.

We have cleaned the drool marks from the piano, the television, and the floors but the memory of him cannot be erased from our hearts. The questions that his life posed, and the answers we found, prevail and compel us to share his story with others who are searching for meaning in similar circumstances.

He lived for twenty-nine years, seven months, and ten days. He was born with a rare chromosome abnormality that caused severe physical and mental handicaps. He grew to be about 5'7" and weighed only one hundred pounds. He was blind in his right eye and had limited vision in the left. He had scoliosis, which caused his spine to curve to the side, and kyphosis, which bent it forward. All of his joints were misaligned with the connecting bones.

He had grand mal seizures. He was prone to upper respiratory infections and pneumonia. Because of a deformity in his neck, his neck muscles alone held his head and spine in alignment. He could not speak beyond a few sounds. He could not feed himself without continual assistance and prompting. We jokingly referred to his gait as "stagger and lurch." He could not chew. He drooled.

His smile lit up his face and endeared him to anyone that noticed. He loved the Muppets; Grover was his favorite. He had a great sense of humor and laughed easily. He only cried twice in his life, once when I scolded him over a minor incident and once, in church, for no reason I could discern. He loved music and always wanted a "dance" partner. He gave tight, bony hugs that conveyed his heart to each recipient. He knew both the upper and lowercase of the alphabet. He used some sign language and also some Bliss Symbols, simple figures that can be combined and recombined for communication by disabled people.

He loved to smell flowers. He was at peace in church and seemed to sense a deepness there. Backing up while riding in a car seemed silly to him and made him laugh. He could be very stubborn if he made up his mind to do something but wasn't allowed to do it. He nodded his head in slow jolts when answering a question in the affirmative or quick, short, defiant shakes to say no. His right index finger was always extended with his thumb tucked between it and the third finger.

He enjoyed drawing circles. He thought whispering was funny. He liked order in his surroundings and routine in his day. He liked dressing up. He disliked the feel of grass on his feet. He often rocked as he sat watching television, nodding rhythmically. He loved sound effects. He loved playing in water, whether in a tub, pan, or pool. He poked soap bubbles with his index finger or formed them into designs. He could spell his name. He loved spinning in circles.

He was happy most of the time.

"For I know the plans I have for you," declares the Lord, "plans to prosper you and not to harm you, plans to give you hope and a future."

JEREMIAH 29:11

For ten years, Rob was our only child. With the exception of hospital stays, a one-week vacation, and a few overnight stays, he lived with us and shared the activities of our lives for every day of his. We were twenty when he was born and fifty when he died. Our hearts were broken on both days. At first, because we weren't wise enough to recognize the blessing that he would be for us, so we grieved over the loss of the life we had dreamed of, the man he should have become. Later, after God had revealed His better plan for us and we had seen the beauty and goodness of His ways over our dreams, we grieved the loss of the life we had come to love and value and cherish.

But the pot he was shaping from the clay was marred in his hands; so the potter formed it into another pot, shaping it as seemed best to him.... "Like clay in the hand of the potter, so are you in my hand."

JEREMIAH 18:4-5

I was unconscious when Rob was born, under the influence of anesthesia, a common medical approach to delivery in 1970. When I woke from the anesthetic and asked where my baby was, I sensed that something was wrong. There had been complications, a doctor told me. My baby had some breathing problems and numerous birth defects. I was overwhelmed by the words and so the doctor sedated me.

Later that evening, Phil and I tried to think positively. There were many things that could be done through medicine, surgery, and education. We would hold on to these positive thoughts. As Phil left to go home, he reminded me that we should just be thankful that nothing was wrong with our son's mind. In fact, Phil mused, "He's probably the smartest little guy you've ever seen." With a hug and a kiss, he said goodnight.

Maternity wards are filled with emotion. When new life emerges into the arms of fathers and mothers who welcome this gift, there is much joy and excitement. But there are many other stories intertwined with these. Young mothers, alone, signing adoption papers but naming the baby as their final act of love; mothers and fathers whose babies have died; mothers and fathers whose babies will live less than normal lives. All these mothers lay in beds side by side. Their stories, emotions, fears, joys, all mixed together. So it was for us. Having no insurance meant that we shared a room with another family. Through the night the nurses brought this mother her infant daughter to feed and tend, but my arms remained empty.

I spent a restless, sleepless night. Our pediatrician came in the next morning to tell me that she was ordering more tests and that a skull X-ray would be taken. Hoping to be reassured,

I asked if anything was wrong with Rob's brain. "We're not sure he even has one," she replied. *Oh, God,* I thought, *How will I tell Phil? Will he stay with me through this? How can we raise a child with so many problems?* Questions and fears began to flood over me. The phone rang and my mother's voice reached out to me. As she had in the past and would in the future, she offered love and faith-filled reassurance that sustained me when I needed it most.

When Phil came that evening after school and work, I told him that our concerns for Rob were even greater than originally thought. He wrapped his arms around me and said, "Then there has to be a reason." I had loved him before these words, but I loved him all over in a new way after these words.

Where does this kind of hope come from? To hope when things look hopeless makes no logical sense. We live in a world that is governed by reason and logic, but there is more to us than flesh and blood and bones. One person's spirit despairs and gives up, another person's spirit hopes and goes on. Everything from then on is shaped from that one choice.

Despair is dark and evil and empty; hope is belief in what you cannot see or prove or know for sure. Hope is a part of faith. Much later in my life I would understand more fully as I read the words from Romans: "Not only so but we also rejoice in our sufferings, because we know that suffering produces perseverance; perseverance, character; and character, hope. And hope does not disappoint us, because God has poured out his love into our hearts by the Holy Spirit, whom he has given us" (Rom 5:3-5).

Beyond Rob's physical difficulties, we needed to know the cause of his impairments. The doctors encouraged us to have

Rob's chromosomes tested since they suspected a genetic defect. They drew blood from him and three long weeks later gave us the results. The cause, it turned out, was unknown but the diagnosis was that he would be severely to profoundly retarded, small for his age, and he would have a short life expectancy extending to his early teens at the latest. Then the doctors suggested that we also receive genetic testing to determine the probability of having more children like Rob.

Once again, a long wait amid many fears but then the tests came back showing that we were not carriers of this anomaly. We were told to institutionalize our son and have another child as soon as possible. We should move on with our young lives and forget this had happened. I can still remember the feelings I had while standing in that little room as three doctors in white coats stood giving their advice and counsel. We were twenty years old and sure of everything we knew nothing about, but the one thing we were most certain about was that we were responsible for this life and Rob needed us. He had a right to our love and tending. God prepared us to be parents by giving us responsible parents. Hardships in their lives showed us that you didn't quit when times got tough. You tried harder.

A man's steps are directed by the Lord. How then can anyone understand his own way?

PROVERBS 20:24

Still we would not have chosen this course for our lives. If the selection process had been different, we would have chosen another baby to hold in our arms. Each time I go to the produce aisle I think of life's choices. We select what looks good to our eyes. We select by what we think we know to be good. A bruised peach might actually taste sweeter once you get past the bruise but we set that one aside.

Our humanness makes us seek perfection. Some seek it beyond themselves, some only seek it within. We all confront the same choices that were presented in the Garden of Eden. Do we trust God's perfection or do we become our own god?

By any human standard, we did not appear to be the best parents for such a child. We were really children ourselves. No person I know would have looked at us and said, "These should be his parents." We had two choices. We could believe that this was just an accident, a random happening, or we could believe that there was some higher purpose involved. To believe in a divine plan, though, meant to believe in a Divine Planner.

But how could this Divine Planner be so cruel? In Sunday school I had memorized the verse that said "God is love." How did love fit into all this? Did God Himself stand outside all that was going on, watching to see which way we'd turn, or had He actually caused our situation to be the way it was? I did not yet understand that I stood in the wrong place to see the answers.

I did not understand Scripture: "'For my thoughts are not your thoughts, neither are your ways my ways,' declares the Lord. 'As the heavens are higher than the earth, so are my ways higher than your ways and my thoughts than your thoughts'" (Is 55:8-9).

I did not understand that this small child would be the instrument God would use to make me examine myself and the world around me, to help me see what was really more important.

I did not understand that God had drawn me closer to Him through this life. From this point on, I would see Him more clearly and more personally with every passing day.

I *did* begin to understand the need to wait on the Lord. At one point I whispered in my heart, "Thy will be done."

~ TWO ~

A gift opens the way for the giver and ushers him into the presence of the great.

PROVERBS 18:16

"Step out and wait," God seemed to be saying. We didn't know what was ahead. We didn't know how any of this would end. We didn't know if we could do it. We didn't know how we would pay for it. Everything seemed impossible.

In such circumstances you can only take care of the moment. And that is what we did. No long-range plans, no master plan: only the moment, at most the day. As God provided for the Israelites in the desert, so He provided for us. Many days seemed endless, though. We carried with us a sense that "a cord of three strands is not quickly broken" (Eccl 4:12) and so we moved from day to day.

To be told by educated, professional people to discard or disregard a life is to be told the standards that society values. To have worth, one must make an accepted contribution, be wanted, be deserving of our investment of time and money. We place a premium on these things, the tangible evidence for our judgments. We can easily defend these values when challenged. But lives that come to us outside the accepted normal package make us look more deeply at the way we judge and the values we hold. What happens if we make crucial decisions at the wrong time, before we have all the facts?

Doesn't a life have to be lived to know its value?

"Step out and learn," God also seemed to be saying. We held fast to the child cradled in our arms and established our course against the flow. Being Rob's parents set us apart from the world. Being set apart creates both isolation and freedom. By embracing a life that was rejected by the world as valueless, we were in uncharted waters. There were no Dr. Spock books to read, and even our parents felt unable to give us advice. They carried their own sorrows and fears for us. The goal of every parent is an independent child, but Rob would always be dependent.

In the early '70s there were few highly visible support groups and fewer educational programs. Public ignorance about special needs children and their parents was widespread. Mental institutions were filled to overflowing and the conditions in them were appalling. Our nation stood on the brink of a major shift in thinking and treatment of mentally and physically handicapped people. At the same time, it was about to legalize abortion in an attempt to diminish the number of such people.

Little did we know that our decision concerning Rob would be the cornerstone of our marriage. By saying "yes" to Rob we were making a deeper commitment to each other and to the love between us. We saw in each other the qualities of compassion, determination, and devotion that were essential for our relationship to grow and endure. This small infant shined God's light on who we were and what He would make of us. Rob's weakness made our marriage stronger and our love deeper. Respect grew between us. By linking our hearts through our silent pledges, we became one in purpose and more secure in the other's love.

Years later, when difficult economic times tested us in a far different way, the importance of doing the right thing again impressed itself on us. Advisors counseled us to walk away from a large business debt rather than claim responsibility and endure personal risk and hardship. How could we turn our back on this, any more than we could on Rob? Decisions throughout our lives were formed by the first one we made, and so it is for all of us.

Genetic testing showed that Rob's life had begun normally but after initial cell divisions something altered the chromosomes. A mutation occurred and part of the twenty-first chromosome was missing. This resulted in a child with many characteristics that are the opposite of Down Syndrome where the twenty-first chromosome has an *additional* piece of genetic material. Such a miniscule alteration, such a profound change for both groups. We found ourselves in awe of the complexity and intricacy of human life and ultimately of its Creator.

Rob's condition intrigued doctors. Genetic research was a growing field of study in the '70s. Numerous hospitals and medical schools asked if Rob could become part of their research. Rob would be poked and biopsied for blood or skin samples, photographed, and tested. His case study was included in a genetic conference in Paris in late August of 1971 and his picture was used in *Pediatrics* in the January/February issue in 1972. He was becoming a contributor simply through his existence. We believed that Rob's life had meaning and purpose even if others only viewed him as a "specimen."

While it is never wrong to pursue knowledge, there are always choices to be made once we have that knowledge.

Doctors could now test babies in the womb to see if they were defective. Mothers and fathers were faced with decisions never before imagined. Ultimately, we are seeking more and more control over our future course. But we see with such limited vision. We only see today.

~ THREE ~

Love never fails. But where there are prophecies, they will cease; where there are tongues, they will be stilled; where there is knowledge, it will pass away. For we know in part and we prophesy in part, but when perfection comes, the imperfect disappears. When I was a child, I talked like a child, I thought like a child, I reasoned like a child. When I became a man, I put childish ways behind me. Now we see but a poor reflection as in a mirror; then we shall see face to face. Now I know in part; then I shall know fully, even as I am fully known.

1 CORINTHIANS 13:8-12

During Phil's senior year in college, he had to prepare a short video presentation for a television documentary class. He decided to present a piece about Rob that combined still black-and-white photos with a compelling voice-over. Time was limited, and between Phil's decision and his deadline, Rob was hospitalized. Many of the photos Phil took were of Rob in the hospital, struggling to survive. Phil titled his essay, "At One Year, He's Three Months." The piece touched many people, and some encouraged Phil to show it to KMOX-TV in St. Louis where he was interning. The Public Affairs Director there decided to include this tape in a larger program about genetic research.

From our first days with him we saw Rob as a fighter and survivor. Even without a voice he seemed to be crying out to live. Many who viewed the television segment began to see him as we saw him. Reaction from friends and family encouraged and motivated us to believe that others could also see that Rob's life had a greater purpose than any of us could imagine. We began feeling the pride that society denied us at his birth. We also sensed a growing responsibility to help others know what we were learning. By opening up our lives to others, we saw that God was using all the events of the past to lead us to greater things in the future. Without our knowing it, love had led to hope and hope was leading to trust.

From the beginning, God used other people to remind us of His faithfulness even when we were unfaithful to Him. One letter that we received following the program on Rob came from Notre Dame College in St. Louis. Sr. Francis Marie Sellmeyer wrote to both KMOX-TV and to us in support of such programming and in support of our efforts with Rob.

She said: "I saw the 'Story of Robbie' the other evening, and was most happy to learn about the research going on which can contribute much toward the birth of normal, healthy children. But my reason for writing to you is to thank you for the tremendous gift of life you have given to Robbie. While it is true that now he cannot do and enjoy all that other children can do and enjoy, it is also true that in the next life, Robbie will be perfectly normal and will enjoy forever a life of unimaginable happiness with God and with you. That future happiness would not be possible without the gift of life which you have given to him; and Robbie will be forever grateful to you and love you for the gift of your love and of life to him. May God bless you and enrich your lives in a special way for all you have shared with Robbie."

~ FOUR ~

Do not consider his appearance or his height.... The Lord does not look at the things man looks at. Man looks at the outward appearance, but the Lord looks at the heart.

1 Samuel 16:7

Many people still view lives such as Rob's as mistakes, accidents, freaks. But judgments based on external conditions are rarely worth much. Rob's outer package was biologically flawed but he had an inner beauty and joy. His life made me rethink my surface judgments and called me to greater discernment.

Years later I realized how much I had learned of God through Rob's life. Greater awareness made me see how flawed I am. The world rejected Rob because of his appearance and condition, just as God could have rejected me when He looked at my sinful state. The love that Jesus poured out through His sacrifice made the difference in how the Father looks at me. Just so, our love made the difference in how we looked at Rob.

But this kind of love had a price, too. We had to get rid of what we wanted for ourselves and concentrate on what Rob needed. All parents do this but parents of special needs children are called to do it—at least initially—for seemingly few rewards and with little support.

I saw this clearly on the first day of Rob's life. In the hospital, no one talked to me about my baby except to inform me of tests he endured. His picture wasn't taken like all the other children who were healthy and normal. The staff didn't encourage me to visit him in the nursery and I wasn't allowed to touch him. Everyone ignored us. Fortunately, neonatal nurseries have changed in the years since. Compassion for the newborn and the parents has replaced some of the fear and isolation. But even then, we believed that contrary to what the doctors said, we could make a difference.

Humanly speaking, the odds were against us. We were both college students, had no insurance, and faced desperate economic conditions. Naturally, many of our decisions were based on money and our need for it. Once I completed my associate's degree, I accepted a secretarial position. Phil worked several part-time jobs and attended school full-time.

Rob was sick most of the time. He was difficult to feed. He did not suck and had to be tube-fed in the beginning. Later, we had to coax and prod him to eat each drop or mouthful. Feeding was tedious and time-consuming. He threw up many entire feedings and we had to feed him again. After numerous disasters with childcare providers, we were blessed to find a nurse working out of her home who gave loving care when we were away. Sleep became a rare commodity, since Rob's night feedings consumed many hours. Each month brought a new crisis or health-related problem.

After a year, I knew that Rob needed his mother home full-time. Somehow we would work through the financial concerns. More than anything else, I didn't want to look back with regret because I was somewhere else when he needed me most.

Phil was completing his bachelor's degree but knew the importance of getting his master's. We had made it through two very difficult years; one more seemed possible. The job market was tight and everyone was looking for a way to be more valuable to an employer. Phil landed a graduate assistantship and we were all three off to Michigan State University.

After settling in, we contacted the local Association for Retarded Citizens (ARC) and discovered there was a school available for Rob. Michigan was one of the country's leaders in special education and had requirements and provisions that far exceeded other states at the time. When we toured the Beekman Center we cried tears of joy. Beekman offered hope for the future. There no one turned away; we were all welcomed. We needed this acceptance as much as Rob did.

Attending school opened up new opportunities and experiences for Rob, but it also exposed him to more illnesses. He seemed to be coming down with something or recovering from something all the time. The uncertainty of his health and his physical needs made employment for me impossible. When he was well, though, I needed something to do with my time so I began to do volunteer work. I helped at the school or at the ARC whenever there was a need. Phil and I got involved in the political and legislative aspects of special education. We helped with petition drives, letter writing, and telephone campaigns seeking improvements on state and national levels.

Rob's needs opened our eyes to the needs of all such children and adults. Our awareness and sensitivity grew as our love had grown for him. Loving Rob had now opened us up to love others in a new way.

~ FIVE ~

*His disciples asked him, "Rabbi, who sinned, this man or his parents, that he was born blind?" "Neither this man nor his parents sinned," said Jesus, **"but this happened so that the work of God might be displayed in his life."***

JOHN 9:2-3, emphasis mine

Rob began having seizures one month before his first birthday. We heard an unusual sound coming from his room late one night and hurried in to find him convulsing. We rushed him to the emergency room. After numerous tests and a spinal tap the doctors concluded that this was just another aspect of Rob's life, which we would have to include in ours. On numerous occasions we had to hospitalize him while the doctors adjusted his medication. Once he had a seizure so severe that the doctors couldn't give him a stronger doze of anticonvulsant for fear of an overdose. We were informed that if the seizure activity didn't stop soon, he would probably have a heart attack. The convulsion subsided and we resumed our lives.

To say we resumed our lives implies that there was no change but each day with Rob felt like a borrowed day and we wanted to make the most of his time with us. He was helping us to see the importance and urgency of each of our days. Without our knowing it, he taught us about stewardship, about how to use fully what God gives us. And he did it all without words, with a smile, and with courage. If he could do it, shouldn't we?

Each hospital visit brought us in contact with people who were confronted daily with life and death. Long days of waiting and hours spent in small rooms opened our eyes to countless people who had nowhere else to go for help. And so they sat patiently, waiting in rooms filled to overflowing with bald heads, bandaged parts, wounded souls.

Why are they so patient, I wondered, when the world is so impatient? People find it hard to wait for the stoplight to turn green, and yet these people, to whom time has the utmost meaning, wait patiently. It occurred to me that the hope that what is damaged can be repaired, that there is an answer, that there is a cure, creates this attitude. The older I got the more I saw that the whole world is really a waiting room. We are all sick or damaged somehow. We all need a cure.

Merely hanging on to life for life's sake seemed empty. There had to be more to all this than simply another day of existence. Providing for the education and social needs of Rob and children like him made us feel like we were doing something of value. But we seemed to be avoiding deeper questions, caught up, as we were, in surface issues.

Rob was baptized on the day he was born. Doctors were not sure that he would live past the first twenty-four hours. The minister who had married us came quickly but hospital policy kept all our relatives away. How God was keeping us even then, when we were so far away from Him. What comfort there was that through the promises for all generations our son would be included. The world might turn its back on him but God wouldn't.

"I have summoned you by name" (Is 43:1)—yes, called you through these parents who have wandered far away from Me. My words, spoken to them through their own baptisms, then in Sunday school classes and catechism and worship and family prayer, now move them back to Me through your life. "You are Mine" (Is 43:1) as they are Mine. Cleansing water, healing words, a new creation, a child of God, and an heir of heaven.

And yet, I ignored the occasional tugs at my conscience to go back to church.

But the tugs got stronger. We felt the need for more in our life, both for Rob and for ourselves. We thought the answer was having more family or doing meaningful things. We set out to make things better. We refinished furniture, painted, papered, shined, polished, volunteered, but nothing filled the void. Rob had come so quickly. We thought that just thinking about having more children would make them a reality. We believed it was up to us to choose the time and place. All of our friends and acquaintances were planning and having families now and a part of us hoped for a way to fit back in. But to our surprise, we were not able to have more children.

To say there was no fear in the idea of another pregnancy would be untrue. Genetic workups on us revealed that our chances for having another child like Rob were miniscule. A part of me felt guilty to want such assurances. I loved Rob and who he was, but I longed for a child I could share myself with more completely and one who would share himself with me. I wanted to see a child grow up, be a teen, an adult, get married, have children.

All I had ever dreamed of being was a mother. For me it was

the ultimate work. Though I ached for the role of motherhood on a level apart from the one that now consumed me, I was also afraid that having another child with handicaps would be more than I could physically and emotionally handle, even though I would never have believed I could handle Rob before I had him.

Trust—and in whom we would place our trust—became issues. We knew that testing would be available during pregnancy, but we both agreed that we could not choose abortion. Once begun, we would accept whatever was to be. Rob's life had taught us the value of such acceptance. We had the mistaken impression that we could control the start of a life but agreed that there were boundaries we could not cross, decisions we would not make, values we could not compromise. "Thou shall not kill," meant just that to us. Without verbalizing it, we both agreed that God would be in control after that. We could go so far and no farther.

But the issue of control and acceptance became a factor. I could not get pregnant. A year passed, and then another. Rob was five when we first decided to expand our family, now he was seven. After Rob was born, I stopped looking at other children and focused only on him. I didn't make comparisons, didn't allow myself to think what he would have been doing "if." We were as different as he was different. Now I wanted to be like other women. Now I wanted what seemed to come so easily to everyone but me. Now I began to look at the ease of movement of children at play; at big, round, seeing eyes; at mothers bending down to explain rules or give guidance. Everything seemed to remind me of what was missing in my life with Rob.

And as Rob had gotten older, as he had become mobile, his differences were more and more obvious. People turned away quickly as we passed in stores. Children pointed and asked loud questions. Other mothers were embarrassed or apprehensive about making contact at the park or in the neighborhood. Again I realized that the first step had to be ours. People would approach us if we were more approachable. There was sympathy, curiosity, and fear behind their actions.

To get close to someone's suffering is to make it part of your own, and which of us purposely chooses suffering? Many of these young mothers wanted only to savor these moments of their lives. Rob was a reminder of other possibilities, of other realities. It was easier, safer to feel a momentary pang of sympathy and move away from the uncomfortable and unfamiliar. It wasn't their fault. We would have to teach others just as we had had to learn. But learning and teaching at the same time was not always easy.

I was aware from the start that it was important to make Rob look approachable. Human nature could be used *for* us as it could be used *against* us. We kept Rob clean and fresh smelling, took care of his hair and his teeth, trimmed his fingernails, made sure his clothes looked right together, shined his shoes, and, years later, shaved him. Simply paying more attention to his physical appearance made a difference in how he was treated by other people. And ultimately it made a difference in how he felt about himself. We would use what we could to make his life as good as it could possibly be.

Still, despite our best efforts many would quickly turn away in disgust. Many wouldn't even try to mask their thoughts, regarding themselves as above our circumstance. I remembered the stories of Jesus that I had learned so long ago, that had been so real to me then but were becoming more so with every passing day. The experiences of Rob's life were drawing me closer to my Savior than I realized.

Later, I would read with new understanding the rejection that Jesus endured for those He loved. "He had no beauty or majesty to attract us to him, nothing in his appearance that we should desire him. He was despised and rejected by men, a man of sorrows, and familiar with suffering. Like one from whom men hide their faces he was despised, and we esteemed him not" (Is 53:2-3). Rob was in good company.

One day, when Rob was quite young, we were shopping in a store. A woman walked over, looked at Rob sitting in the cart and said, "I don't know what you did but you certainly must have sinned." She turned and walked away. Her words ring in my head today as they did when she spoke them. My first response was one of anger: "Lady, you're born, but you're not dead yet," I immediately thought. As the years have passed and I rethink her statement I wonder if she wasn't an angel reminding me of where all this started.

Was it necessary to find a specific sin responsible for Rob's problems or was it more important to see the condition of us all in this sin-filled world? We are a people more and more apt to look for somewhere to place blame and find fault, as long as it is outside ourselves. The flaws in Rob were no greater than the flaws in me, only more visible to the naked eye.

Many times I felt trapped by the world's vision. Phil and I took many snapshots of Rob from the time we brought him home from the hospital. For reasons known only to him, the hospital photographer had not taken Rob's picture during his stay in the nursery. Because I shared a room with another mother who peered over the photos of her newborn daughter, I was deeply hurt. "They think he's too ugly for a picture," I thought.

Over the next several months, a local franchise photography studio called me numerous times to inform me of package deals but all I could remember was the reaction of the first photographer. I was too hurt to subject myself to another reaction like that so I was grateful that we were too poor to afford this luxury. Still they continued to call until one day I lost patience and blurted out that our baby had birth defects and to please stop calling. They stopped, but I still struggled with the whole idea of professional photographs of Rob.

Honestly, part of me *was* ashamed. My pride *was* a factor. This child would never win any beauty prizes. I had always valued beauty. I knew that what I saw in Rob went beyond anything a still photo could record. I had seen his determination, his courage, his positive attitude when confronted with seemingly insurmountable obstacles. But I could also see what others saw, his weakness, his vulnerability, his handicaps. I knew we were all a product of God's hand but I was still trying to fit into the world's view. How could I see clearly?

Joy, the nurse who provided day care, had two children of her own. She looked after Rob in such a loving and tender way. Joy had been caring for Rob for about six months when Christmas rolled around. One day, she gave us a flat, rectangular shaped package, a present that went beyond anything she could have known. As I opened it, tears filled my eyes, and my heart softened. In my hands was a picture of a boy dressed in a red vest with a slight smile, one hand raised as if to say "hi."

There was his first professional picture. There was my boy. There was my son. It is one of my most treasured pictures of him to this day, not because of what is seen in the picture but because of what is not seen that I know in my heart. Beauty is in the heart of the beholder.

~ SIX ~

See, it is I who created the blacksmith who fans the coals into flame and forges a weapon fit for its work.

ISAIAH 54:16

As we reached our late twenties, we were finally getting on top of all of the financial burdens that we had carried since Rob's birth. But there were many setbacks. Fresh out of school, Phil had taken a teaching position at a community college in the St. Joseph–Benton Harbor area of Michigan. The job market was tight. His degree in mass communications positioned him for a job in the television industry but there were no jobs available. We could not be picky; teaching English and speech would have to do.

Several months after Phil took the job, all of the teachers went out on strike. Both sides were locked into feelings from the past that we did not share. We were in the middle. Being in the middle causes a person to be mindful of the consequences of a move in any direction. We could not move against either and felt alienated by both. The school fired the entire faculty, replacing them with other teachers. The courts upheld the action—strikes by teachers were illegal. Other schools would strike successfully despite the same illegality, gaining benefits we could only dream of, but we had to move on. Phil worked as a carpenter's assistant for nine months, learning a trade that he would use the rest of his life. Meanwhile, he continued to send out resumes, go on job interviews, and hope for a job that would use his education and provide for our future. I took care of other people's children and sewed and ironed to make a few extra dollars to get us through.

And make it we did. Phil took an entry-level copywriter's job with WOOD-TV in Grand Rapids, Michigan. We now had the first real security that we had known since living in our parents' homes. With the security, the longing for another child grew stronger with every passing day.

Though the journey had been a rocky one, we met wonderful people along the way. Each move brought new friendships to our lives and brought Rob into the lives of others as well. At Michigan State, we met couples in married student housing who have remained our friends ever since. Fondue dinners, exercise classes, anytime get-togethers made us feel part of something bigger than ourselves.

After our move to the St. Joseph area, we became close friends with one of Rob's teachers and her husband. Jan and Milo filled our lives with encouragement and laughter. They helped us move from St. Joseph to Grand Rapids. We had weekends filled with roaring fires, delicious high-calorie meals, and nonstop talking. And when Phil's job required a trip to California, Jan volunteered her babysitting services. We were off for our first real vacation.

It wasn't easy to leave Rob behind but Jan had cared for him in the classroom. I was confident that she knew him as I knew him. After writing down a detailed schedule, complete with doctors, family, and hotel telephone numbers, we said our good-byes. On our return, Jan gave us a journal that she wrote about their adventures during our absence. We laughed as we read about Rob removing flowers from a vase and drinking the water when he was thirsty and Jan didn't move fast enough for him. We chuckled as Jan revealed her new understanding of the balancing act that constituted life with Rob.

Reading it years later, though, I was struck by one story in particular. Jan is not a believer. No kinder, more loving, more decent, more giving person could you find, but in our religious discussions she reminded me that "If you believe, no words are necessary; if you don't believe, no words are possible." Still, Rob had the power to bring this woman to prayer.

We had always said bedtime prayers with Rob even when we weren't saying them for ourselves. As I had done with my sister every night before sleep, so I did with my son. On his first night under Jan's supervision, Rob folded his hands. In her journal, Jan wrote: "I tucked Rob in and was getting ready to leave and noticed Rob was folding his hands. *Aha,* I thought. I asked if Mom said prayers and Rob smiled, so I said, 'God bless Mom.' Rob's smile got bigger so I figured I was on the right track. Next came, 'God bless Daddy, and Grandma and Grandpa Bandy, and Grandma and Grandpa Pilgrim.' By this time Rob was praying with me. I was trying desperately to remember Trish's name [Rob's aunt], and failing miserably, so I asked Rob, 'Who else, Robbie?' and he began pounding on his chest. So we finished with a rousing, 'God bless Robbie!'"

We were aware that Rob's life opened up possibilities that were otherwise closed. This was especially true within our own spiritual walk. From the beginning, God was at work through Rob's life to bring us closer to Him. I had been a believer from childhood, never doubting my eternal security. I knew that the price had been paid for my sins. Thus saved by grace, I then erroneously thought I could live my life in whatever way seemed acceptable to me. God's guidelines were a foundation block, but I conveniently separated my beliefs from the details of my daily walk. This was not my church's theology but it was my theology.

Phil's drifting had been more dramatic than my own. Raised and schooled in the church, he had reached a point of real doubt in the reality of God. He studied philosophy and other religions but these only clouded his mind and lured him into an intellectualism that mocked the very idea of an all-knowing, all-powerful, all-saving God. We were ships without rudders, steadily heading off course. But God was drawing us back to Him through that which was dearest to us: Rob and the desire for more children.

The daily challenges and the forces at work in our lives not only moved us to deeper things, they also brought times of pure delight. We appreciated what we had. The love we shared between us was a rare commodity in an increasingly disposable world. We held on to each other and discovered the strength that comes from unity of purpose.

Memories of those years come back to us not as a sorrow but as a blessing. There were even times when we felt like any other parent. One summer after we moved to Grand Rapids, we rented a log cabin on a lake. For one week the three of us had the world to ourselves. Phil was determined to introduce Rob to the outdoor life. He insisted on getting him up early one morning so that the two of them could take a rowboat out and fish. Rob seemed to wonder about the urgency of the early wake-up call but went along with it.

After as quick a breakfast as he could muster, Rob went off with Phil on their adventure. The sun was just peeking over the horizon. I stood watching them walk off thinking what a good man I had married. By the way he was walking, I could see that Rob was excited. Life jackets on, into the boat they climbed. I heard a slight squeal from Rob as Phil pushed off and began rowing. Then it started. The sound rose and with every echo came the next with more fury—Rob's feet stomping gleefully on the bottom of the metal boat, waking the entire community of vacationers. They didn't find any fish but the memory of the two of them in the middle of that lake will last my lifetime.

Through every friendship and every experience, we seemed to be questioning, considering, maturing in those "deeper things." God nudged us along at a pace that encouraged the next step, never too fast, never too slow. At just the right time a woman of deep faith became my friend. She had four children. My desire for a family continued to grow as I watched them interact with one another. I was convinced that much was missing in my life. God continued to speak to me through the lives of other Christians, drawing me toward a closer walk with Him. I began to feel a spiritual longing, but rather than confront my real need, I focused on my physical needs and my emptiness.

Medical intervention seemed our only option if we were to have another child. We began the walk down the infertility trail. This included medical exams for both of us, temperature charts, blood tests, cervical biopsies, fertility drugs, laparoscopy, and surgery for endometriosis. Finally, joy of all joys, I became pregnant. But we held this child only in our hearts, never in our arms. After only twelve weeks, I miscarried. We had chosen the name Christina if our baby was a daughter. Chromosome tests revealed that this baby was indeed a girl with normal chromosomes. The doctors advised us to try again.

> *When I tried to understand all this, it was oppressive to me till I entered the sanctuary of God.*
>
> PSALM 73:16-17

> *I will take refuge in the shadow of your wings until the disaster has passed. I cry out to God Most High, to God, who fulfills his purpose for me.*
>
> PSALM 57:1-2

I had never known such emptiness. Desire gave way to depression and despair. Many days I cried uncontrolled tears. One such day I realized that I had to will myself to stop or I'd be lost in my grief. Looking for some kind of distraction, I picked up one of the textbooks that Phil had used when teaching. I opened it and began reading. The words struck deep inside me.

Under the heading "Winter Light," I read:

> Her dream began with winter darkness. Out of this darkness came a great hand, fisted. It was a man's hand, powerful and hollowed by shadows in the wells between bones and tendons. The fist opened and in the long plain of the palm lay three small pieces of coal. Slowly the hand closed, causing within the fist a tremendous pressure.

The pressure began to generate a white heat and still it increased. There was a sense of weighing, crushing time.

She seemed to feel the suffering of the coal with her own body, almost beyond the point of being borne. At last she cried out to the hand, "Stop it! Will you never end it! Even a stone cannot bear to this limit ... even a stone...!" After what seemed like too long a time for anything molecular to endure, the torments in the fist relaxed. The fist turned slowly and very slowly opened. Diamonds, three of them! Three clear and brilliant diamonds, shot with light, lay in the good palm. A deep voice called to her, "Deborah!" and then, gently, "Deborah, this will be you."

God came to me and held me that day through the words of an unknown author. I needed Him in my life but I didn't know where to look. I saw that my greatest needs could never be found anywhere outside of His "good palm."

Years later I would understand more clearly as I read in Scripture:

Endure hardship as discipline; God is treating you as sons. For what son is not disciplined by his father? If you are not disciplined (and everyone undergoes discipline), then you are illegitimate children and not true sons. Moreover, we have all had human fathers who disciplined us and we respected them for it. How much more should we submit to the Father of our spirits and live!

Our fathers disciplined us for a little while as they thought best; but God disciplines us for our good, that we may share in his holiness. No discipline seems pleasant at the time, but painful. Later on, however, it produces a harvest of righteousness and peace for those who have been trained by it.

HEBREWS 12:7-11

~ SEVEN ~

Deep calls to deep in the roar of your waterfalls; all your waves and breakers have swept over me.

PSALM 42:7

My sister gave birth to her second son and asked me to be his godmother. It was a privilege and an honor. I made the baptismal outfit as my gift to this beautiful, healthy baby. It felt good to be a part of such a wonderful new beginning but my heart ached and the hurt was deep. I wasn't sure I would ever recover from the wound I felt over our inability to have more children.

God was guiding the steps, though, and in the sermon that baptismal Sunday, I heard His voice again as clearly as if He were standing next to me. "Accept My plan. Let go and accept My way." I felt myself give in and in my heart I again said "yes" to what I didn't understand.

We had done everything we could humanly do to make *our* will be done, now we could only wait on the Lord. My mother sent me a note with a quote that said, "If you have a wounded heart, touch it as little as you would an injured eye. There are only two remedies for the suffering of the soul: Hope and Patience."

When we are low in spirit, we look for ways to rise above the circumstances. Sometimes our solutions seem somewhat vague to an onlooker, sometimes they are crystal clear. When we were looking for other sources of fulfillment, we considered getting a pet. Several years before the miscarriage, we took Rob to the Humane Society so that he could see the dogs there. He completely refused to even look at a dog. Instead, he pushed and pointed us in the direction of the cats.

Rob had always loved pictures of cats. He even had a sound for them and later learned the sign for them. He loved the feeling of their fur, but often insisted on rubbing them the wrong way. A cat would never work, I thought. He needs a dog. But Rob would have no part of it so we left the Humane Society animal-less.

On the day before Rob's ninth birthday, Phil called from work. A stray cat had been living at the TV station for a week and he wanted to bring it home for the weekend. We didn't have to keep it, he explained, just try it for the weekend. She was an ugly cat, white with patches of black in all the wrong places. She was fully grown and I knew no one would choose her if she went to the Humane Society. It somehow seemed fitting for her to stay with us. Rob was thrilled. Within a few weeks, she escaped only to come home very dirty and tired. We later realized that Scraps would be a mother in the spring. *How is it possible,* I thought, *that even this animal can do what I am unable to do?* Sure enough, Scraps had four beautiful kittens and in so doing brought hope and joy in the gift of life. If an ugly cat could do it, maybe I could too.

Why are you downcast, O my soul? Why so disturbed within me? Put your hope in God, for I will yet praise him, my Savior and my God.

PSALM 42:5

Within the year I was pregnant again. We counted down the weeks with a mixture of joy and anxiety. I began to spot, and fear came rushing over us. I wanted this child. I wanted to do everything I could to MAKE this child happen. My submission to God's way surely couldn't mean the end of this life, too. My doctor suggested injections that might sustain the pregnancy. He was quick to remind me that if they worked we might be sustaining an abnormal fetus. We had never thought of ourselves as risk takers but that's what we became. The pregnancy continued and after the first trimester, everything progressed normally. I began to dream again, to believe in God's all surpassing goodness no matter what the outcome of this pregnancy. I began to go to church again. And miracle of miracles, Phil came too.

On March 1, 1980, on my due date, Rob became a brother. No words could express the emotion, no joy I'd ever known was as immense. God delivered to us a daughter with two round, wise eyes. I felt His presence in the delivery room and saw His hand in the gift of this child. He knew our need and He gave us His reassurance and His love in this beautiful bundle. We named her Elisabeth Grace—God's promise, God's blessing—for that is what she was to us. In her baby book I wrote: "That which was once empty is now full."

On her baptismal day, just eight days after she was born, the Gospel lesson reminded us that we should always keep in mind how close we had come to dismissing God from our lives. We saw what the consequences of that could have been.

The reading was from Luke. "A man had a fig tree, planted in his vineyard, and he went to look for fruit on it, but did not find any. So he said to the man who took care of the vineyard,

'For three years now I've been coming to look for fruit on this fig tree and haven't found any. Cut it down! Why should it use up the soil?' 'Sir,' the man replied, 'leave it alone for one more year, and I'll dig around it and fertilize it. If it bears fruit next year, fine! If not, then cut it down'" (Lk 13:6-8).

Both Phil and I were aware that God had given us more time and more opportunities to know Him and serve Him. We felt an urgency to make up for all the time we'd lost in our wanderings.

Every addition to a family enlarges the range and scope of each person's life. We understood that this new life would take us down paths that Rob had not been able to journey. His contribution would be passed on in a whole new way and would reach into places he himself would never go. We were rejuvenated.

Overnight, other mothers viewed me as a first-time mother. I was finally one of them even though I had been one of them for ten years, through times of care and concern, heartache and joy. Now I would see what motherhood was really like, they seemed to be saying as I was invited for coffee or to neighborhood gatherings. My years before somehow didn't count; only now did they perceive me as real. But I knew the significance of the previous years, and if they would take the time to know me now they, too, would learn. We would each gain understanding for the other. It was as if I could actually hear the opening of doors.

~ EIGHT ~

My life seemed perfect, filled with new purpose and new direction both physically and spiritually. Contentment and peace flooded over me, replacing sorrow and emptiness. Rob's life even had renewed meaning for me as we looked forward to sharing him with his sister who would see him as we saw him.

Rob continued to grow and thrive in spite of occasional setbacks due to illness. We were involved in his schooling. We continued to believe that we could make a difference in his future if we encouraged his development. Rob loved it when we read to him. When we asked him to find objects in picture books, we were amazed by what he actually understood. It was a real challenge, though, to find activities that reached Rob and led him in meaningful directions. We, along with his teachers, tried to surmount the space between what we thought Rob was capable of understanding and what his limitations allowed. We were all confined by his lack of language and severe physical limitations. Still we tried to move forward.

Each step in Rob's life required many mini-steps and much repetition. He had not learned to suck until he was two years old. At the time, we were ready to get rid of the adapted bottle but when he started sucking we decided to continue with that method a while longer. We thought that this stage of oral development might be necessary or helpful to the development of language. Rob did not walk until he was four years old. He was not toilet trained through the night until he was eleven. Consistent, repetitive, diligent routines were crucial for any improvement. He had to be reminded to swallow to lessen the drooling. Teaching him to brush his teeth, feed, and dress himself required years of work. We never asked ourselves if it was worth it, there was simply no other way.

It never crossed my mind that I should find more important things to do with my time. Rob had been given to us and we would care for him. But his growth required daily vigilance.

Years earlier, I read Doris Lund's book, *Eric,* about her son Eric and his battle with leukemia. I had seen striking similarities between her feelings and my own. To some, it might seem strange for me to relate so clearly to a mother of a normal young man battling a disease. But for me there was a very real comparison. For all the fighting Eric did, the outcome was inevitable. Some would consider the fighting a waste. For all the education or training or love or will to achieve, the outcome for Rob would not be a college degree. So why spend the time? Reading that book, I knew more than ever before that it's how we live that's important. Standards of achievement vary from person to person but the courage to try was as much a part of Rob's life as it was of Eric Lund's.

Doris Lund wrote, "And so, as in a shipwreck or other large-scale disaster, when life came down to basics, the things that counted were bravery, humor, and the will to live." Rob's life was full of basics.

Over the years we had come to know teachers as professional, dedicated, caring people. Occasionally, teachers fresh out of college, looking to make a name for themselves, hoped to revolutionize working with the handicapped.

Overall, though, each person we met was committed to the advancement of each individual student. Everyone had one goal: To help each child live the fullest life possible.

Finding ways to help Rob communicate became an overriding concern. It was obvious that he knew more than he could express. How could we open more areas of expression for him so that he could communicate what he knew? We attempted sign language but dismissed it except for a few simple signs that Rob used the rest of his life. Next, we tried Bliss Symbols, named for their inventor Charles Bliss. To everyone's surprise, these abstract drawings made sense to Rob and in one month he learned thirty-two of them. But his physical limitations made it difficult for him to carry and use them. We made a walletlike book that we attached by a strap to his belt loop. But someone had to pull it out, turn the pages, wait for Rob's response and put it back. Rob would walk around with the book swinging and swaying, looking as if he had been on a leash and made a quick getaway.

Each method seemed to offer hope but in the end, each frustrated Rob. None more than minimally advanced his ability to express himself. Over the years we came to understand his body language and were able to see his wants and needs through that.

Drooling was another major problem in Rob's life. He soaked his clothing and in the Michigan winters we worried about his health. Long bus rides home in wet clothing contributed to chills and colds. We sent changes of clothes to school and with the help of dedicated staff we were able to keep him dry most of the time. On days when he was unusually tired or coming down with something, he became a fountain. We had to wash his winter coat every other day to keep it fresh and sanitary. On especially heavy days, he wore a hand towel specially made with Velcro fasteners.

Always conscious of socially acceptable behavior, we wondered if there was some way to conquer this problem. We learned there was a procedure that would limit drooling in children like Rob and decided to find out more about it. We made an appointment hoping that there might be a way to provide him with a more normal life in this area.

The operation would mean removing his salivary glands and creating a dry mouth. While the operation would cure one problem, we questioned whether it was in Rob's best interest for all his tomorrows. How uncomfortable would it be to have a dry mouth all the time? What would happen to his teeth over time? Would I want this done to me? In the end we decided against the operation, choosing to wait and hope that time would change what we were afraid to alter through surgical intervention.

Heavy responsibilities come to those who care for those who cannot care for themselves. We never knew what Rob wanted outside of his simplest needs. We had the ability to make decisions that would alter his life forever. With that power came the responsibility to make decisions based not on our convenience, but on his best interest.

During Rob's first year of life, he had numerous infections in his blind eye. We took him to an ophthalmologist who wrote in a report: "The right eye could be improved cosmetically at a later age by placing a prosthetic shell in the cul-de-sac. The shell would include a likeness of an iris, pupil, conjunctival blood vessels, and so on."

But Rob's face was beginning to look very deformed by the time he was seven years old. Although we had been advised to wait until he was older, we wanted to correct this abnormality. A doctor in Southfield, Michigan, was able to help. He prepared Rob for his eventual prosthesis through the use of a small plastic device that stretched the muscles. He said that if we had waited until Rob was a teenager, as we had been told to do, his muscles would have atrophied so that a prosthesis would have been impossible.

Numerous six-hour trips to Southfield from Grand Rapids over the course of a year with yearly follow-ups produced incredible results. Cosmetically, the difference for Rob was phenomenal. Over the years we had many laughs while going on "eye hunts" or discovering the prosthetic eye in some unexpected place. For the most part, though, Rob kept the prosthesis in and seemed to be aware of and pleased by his changed appearance. He loved to look in a mirror.

What to change and what to be content with became elements of all our days with Rob. As the years passed, we saw that despite all our efforts and all our encouragement, Rob would never reach another level of development. On the other hand, we were convinced that our constant encouragement and support helped him achieve the level he had attained. We always had expectations for Rob but it became clear that we should accept certain realities in order to fully enjoy and respect his nature and personality. Knowing when to push or demand and when to give in were issues we faced with him just as all parents face with their children. He would be the first one to let us know if we were being unreasonable and he would do so in no uncertain terms.

After learning to walk at the age of four, two basic goals remained foremost for Rob. We always held on to the hope that he would learn to feed himself and use the toilet independently. These were essential skills that would enable him to have a life outside a total care setting. Even if he remained in our home for the rest of his life, lack of these skills would complicate all our normal routines and activities. No matter what level he would finally reach, the effort to attain these goals seemed worth it because they would enhance his life (and ours) on a daily basis.

Whenever Rob made progress and we congratulated him, he would smile his broadest smile and drink in the compliments. He truly wanted to please. After eleven years he was trained through the night. Because he could not fully manipulate buttons, snaps, and zippers, especially under emergency conditions, he never achieved total independence. But his days were more comfortable once he was on a schedule and complied. With only a few exceptions (for example, he loved chocolate milk, graham crackers, and cookies) he never seemed to care whether he ate or not. This area remained under our supervision and direction for all his years.

As there were physical challenges, so also there were spiritual challenges connected to life with Rob. We lived in a community composed mainly of believers in decision theology which relies on the conscious acceptance of Jesus as Lord and Savior for eternal security. In this setting, our thoughts and beliefs on infant baptism and the kingdom of grace were regularly questioned.

Phil and I had been born and raised in communities of faith that embraced infant baptism. We were naively surprised by the thoughts and beliefs of Christian friends and coworkers who found our views misguided. Their questions and comments drove us deeper into the study of God's Word and promises. We could not disagree with them regarding conversion experiences since the Bible clearly supported such occurrences. But in the area of infant baptism we found ourselves at odds.

For many of our sincere Christian friends and acquaintances, our belief defied reason and their understanding of Scripture. For them, making a personal decision for Christ was the goal for every human being. For them, Rob's very existence posed questions that they could not answer for me.

Did Rob, and all others like him, including all newborns and stillborns and miscarried children, stand outside God's grace because they could not understand God with their minds? Did Rob's salvation depend on his ability to comprehend God's words? Did the limits of his intellect determine the limits of God's grace? Did he have to understand God to be a member of God's family? Was the kingdom designed to keep the Robs of this world out or was Rob designed to show us the width and depth of the kingdom's grace? The more I studied, the more I saw a God who covered Rob's imperfections (and mine). It was God's acceptance of us that was important, not our acceptance of Him.

Through study of the Old Testament, for example, I saw that circumcision was performed on every male on the eighth day of life as a sign of the covenant agreement between that child and God. "You are mine and I am yours," God said. There was no evidence that each child understood what was happening. Grace was happening, unmerited, unexplained, undeserved. Parents were to be faithful in their obedience to this command of God.

But salvation was not dependent on human obedience. God Himself showed His mercy to children even when their parents disobeyed. He said: "And the little ones that you said would be taken captive, your children who do not yet know good from bad—they will enter the land. I will give it to them and they will take possession of it" (Dt 1:39). Were these blessings only physical, earthly blessings? Was God not always leading us to spiritual blessings through all His teachings?

Following God's instruction into the New Testament, I saw how Jesus included children by saying, "Make disciples of *all* nations, baptizing them in the name of the Father and of the Son and of the Holy Spirit, and teaching them to obey everything I have commanded you" (Mt 28:19-20, emphasis mine). Water connected with the Word of God through the power of the Holy Spirit changed hearts and produced disciples.

Further work of the Spirit through instruction of the Word deepened the relationship begun by God in baptism. God promised to be faithful to His Word to complete the good work already begun.

Time and again, the New Testament showed me that entire households of the early church were baptized (Stephanas' household in 1 Corinthians 1:16; Lydia's household in Acts 16:15; the jailer at Philippi's household in Acts 16:33; Crispus' household in Acts 18:8). "You are all sons of God through faith in Christ Jesus, for all of you who were baptized into Christ have clothed yourselves with Christ" (Gal 3:26-27) ... "the promise is for you and your children" (Acts 2:39).

The power of God is in the Word of God. The power of circumcision, the power of the Ark of the Covenant, the power of the bronze serpent, the power of the blood of Passover lay beyond the physical elements. Yet the elements themselves, when connected to God's Word, conveyed blessings and forgiveness. God said do *this* and *this* will happen. So too, we believed that God would be faithful to His promise of cleansing through baptism.

We know faith comes by hearing, not necessarily by understanding. The power is God's, the work is God's. Can a child in the womb not hear? Did John the Baptist not leap in his mother's womb when Mary came to Elizabeth? Is the work of the Holy Spirit confined only to the mature and intelligent? Indeed it is God who grants our minds the ability to understand: "The Lord has not given you a mind that understands or eyes that see or ears that hear" (Dt 29:4). "Who then can be saved?" asked the disciples. Jesus looked at them and said, "With man this is impossible, but with God all things are possible" (Mt 19:26, see Mk 10:27).

Just as Noah and his family were saved by water, Rob's baptism now saved him. This was "not the removal of dirt from the body, but the pledge of a good conscience toward God. It saves you by the resurrection of Jesus Christ" (1 Pt 3:21).

We saw Rob's baptism not as a superstition or ritual or ceremony or tradition, but as the work of Jesus for the salvation of Rob's soul. We were confident that through it God would be faithful to His promises and the eternal hope that we had for our child. God promised that this hope would not disappoint us.

I believed these promises because I knew they were true in my life. I had never known a time when I had not believed in

God. I had known times when I had strayed from Him, when I had tested Him, when I was too busy for Him, when I had disobeyed Him, but I had never known a day without Him. Washed, justified, sanctified: herein was our hope and peace for Rob and ourselves.

Again and again God had led us to search for Him through the very existence of Rob. The challenges of each day remained, whether physical or spiritual, but through these we began to see how God was "growing us," how He patiently nurtured us toward maturity, how He used us in the lives of others.

~ NINE ~

There were weary days though, days when we collapsed into bed wondering if we could physically do it again tomorrow. Days of stark reality always followed, reminding us of other possibilities. In one year, shortly after Elisabeth was born, four of Rob's schoolmates died. We knew that life was a precious gift. We treasured Rob's.

He was easy to treasure. His smile was so genuine. He loved music and learned to hum "This Old Man" when he was seven. He would pull albums out of their covers and place the record on the turntable. Whenever we visited Phil's parents, Rob headed straight for the organ where he spent the longest time creating "songs." Phil taught him the beginning of "Three Blind Mice" and it became a regular request. Some attempts to find ways for him to participate in music backfired, however. After doing clapping rhythms one week, he clapped through every hymn in church the following Sunday.

And he had a pure heart. To test his ability to distinguish his own coat from ours, we threw them all on the floor and told him to find his. He staggered over to the pile, bent down slowly, carefully pulled out my coat and wearing the biggest smile possible, walked it over to me first. At times like these he would be so delighted with himself.

His innocence and pure heart caught us off guard at times. When he was about five years old, his Uncle Dave took him for a walk to stretch his legs. When the two of them came back,

Rob was carrying a white Fuji (spider) mum. They had stopped at a florist shop and Dave had told Rob to pick out any flower he wanted. To Dave's surprise, Rob chose the one that looked like an explosion held together in perfect order. How much like Rob this flower was. He beamed as he handed his choice to me. I can still see his face.

On yet another day, he and his classmates and teachers were out enjoying an early spring day. The teachers encouraged each child to pick or smell flowers. Some found dandelions, some forsythia, and each received a small bouquet. Most of them left their flowers lying on the ground as they were sidetracked by some new distraction. When I went to the bus to bring him inside our house, there sat Rob still holding tightly to his bouquet, eager to share it with Mom. The bus ride had been over forty minutes long. The forsythia sat on our windowsill for two weeks.

Rob's personality bloomed at school, too. His teachers and I sent a notebook back and forth to keep each other informed about our concerns or details that Rob could not communicate. We recorded and exchanged news of how well he had eaten, or if he was out of sorts on any particular day, or if he had fallen, or accomplished a goal like using scissors, or learned more sign language, or if we had suspicions of a change in health.

One such note came home saying that on that day they had played a shoe game, but that Rob, being very particular and protective about his feet, had adamantly refused to play. He didn't want to take his shoes off. So his teacher put him in a corner while all the others played the game. When they were done, he came over to the teacher with both shoes in his hand. He had untied them and taken them off all by himself, a tremendous display of effort and determination on his part. She reported that he was as proud of his accomplishment as she was of his change of heart.

Rob had again been included in a television segment. The piece was called "No Institution for Robbie." The purpose of the program was to encourage and inform new parents of handicapped children. We hoped that increased awareness would benefit all such children. Around this time, the Association for Retarded Citizens made a film for national distribution that we also participated in. The film was called "Readin' and Writin' Ain't Everything" and we were told that President Ford, Mrs. Ford, and the president's advisor on mental retardation all viewed the film before it was released.

We had also accepted several speaking engagements over the years. Never quite comfortable with being spokesmen, yet never reluctant to share Rob with others, we accepted one such request from Calvin College. We addressed a group of special education students. Later we received a letter from the instructor that said: "The insights and powerful feelings which you shared gave us a much clearer understanding of the dynamics of having a retarded child. The students in my class will soon be working with other children like Robbie and with their families. You have helped ensure that these interactions will be more compassionate and insightful. Thank you for filling a crucial need." Again Rob's life was taking on meaning beyond our lives.

With all of Rob's challenges, we would have given anything to keep him from more hardship or suffering. Despite all our efforts and sometimes because of them, Rob's mobility and encounters with the world brought numerous accidents. Once, he pulled a coffeepot over on himself after I moved the pot to what I thought was a safer location. As I carried him past the pot, he caught the cord with an outstretched hand. Good judgment failed me and I pulled his shirt off, thinking I should get the heat off him as quickly as possible. His skin came off with the shirt. He spent nearly three weeks in the hospital, his skin turning black from the silver nitrate treatments.

There had been any number of cuts, bruises, and stitches because his awkward gait caused him to stumble. And then one day in early October, when Elisabeth was three years old, I got a call from the school principal saying that there had been an accident. Rob had fallen into the school pool without a life jacket and was in critical condition. When they found him, he wasn't breathing but his heart was still beating. He was on his way to the hospital. I quickly found a neighbor to take care of Elisabeth. We were a one-car family so I picked up Phil from work and we went to the hospital together.

Rob was indeed in trouble. His color wasn't good. The doctors were concerned about infection in his lungs. The water in the pool was kept at a very warm temperature for therapeutic reasons, since most of the children had spastic limbs. Rob again made the local nightly TV news and the press. After a little more than a day in ICU, the doctors put him in a regular room.

In that room, a six-year-old girl with long blonde hair lay in a coma. A car had hit her on her way to school and there was little hope for her recovery. Again we were reminded of how fragile this life is and how thankful we were to have yet another extension of Rob's.

We were surprised by people's reactions following the accident. Many advised us to sue the school for negligence since Rob was not wearing a life jacket and was not adequately supervised. While we agreed that both of these facts were true, we also believed that there had been no overt attempt to harm Rob, only a mistake in judgment and procedures. The teachers and aides responsible for Rob's class were deeply troubled by Rob's condition. These were people who cared for him physically in all the same ways that we did. They, too, were touched by him emotionally. More important, they were genuinely sorry for the accident.

Could we say that we had never made a mistake in judgment regarding his well-being? Would we want to be punished beyond our own guilt over such an error? Could one oversight cancel out all our times of doing what was best for him? Why then should we judge them differently than we wanted to be judged?

The school made changes in policies regarding the pool area and instruction. Students wore life jackets from then on. Rob had again been used to make this place a safer place for all who would come after him. He never suffered any long-term effects of the incident and we again had reason for thanks.

~ TEN ~

Ironically, it was Rob's slowness in learning that helped us fully appreciate Elisabeth's quickness. We marveled and delighted in every stage of development and over every word she spoke, even over the way her body was put together and worked. What had taken Rob years to accomplish or even to attempt, took her only days or months. We had Rob to thank for the sense of wonder that we felt every day with her. Our deep appreciation and awareness for these blessings came from having had Rob first. Without his life, we might easily have taken a normal child for granted. But we were able to savor the joy because of the insight we received from Rob's life.

From her earliest days, Elisabeth's eyes were opened to much that others never know. She often came with me to Rob's school, watched her brother compete in Special Olympics, saw the reactions of others toward him in the neighborhood, community, and church. We are never sure how these experiences will affect a child. Would she look for ways to get away from the connection or would she treasure the memories and realize their importance?

One day when Phil was painting the house, in the summer of Elisabeth's third year, she said, "When Robbie gets older and bigger and he can talk, then he can paint the house too." Phil said, "No, Robbie will never grow up like that." To which Elisabeth said, "That makes me sad." By the time she was four she would introduce Rob to her friends by saying, "This is my big brother Rob. He's retarded. He can't talk, but he sings pretty songs."

When we thought life was the best that it possibly could be, it got better. We were pregnant again! Then after eight short weeks, I miscarried. Reminders of old sorrows, as well as thanksgiving for the lives we had been blessed with, deepened and strengthened us. In less than six months I was pregnant again, only to lose that child as well. A sense of wonder filled us that any pregnancy ended in a live child. We began to believe that we had all the family God intended us to have. While we were willing to accept this plan, we still hoped for another child.

Then came another pregnancy. After a little trouble in the first trimester, everything progressed normally. I was more relaxed as my due date approached than I had been with Elisabeth, but fears sometimes rose up. People stared less with this pregnancy. Elisabeth's presence seemed to calm their judgment. One week past my due date we were still waiting. One and one half weeks past, we were still waiting. I had stress tests and days later, Bryan Christopher arrived two weeks later than expected. When he did, he came in spectacular fashion and I barely made it to the hospital for delivery.

His name means "strength, honor, courage," "bearing Christ." That was what we hoped for in this new life. Our faith was growing daily through reading and studying the Word, through weekly worship, through the gift of the Sacrament, and through fellowship with Christian friends. There was a growing, consuming need to share this knowledge with and through our children.

We began to look at all the areas of our lives to see how each measured up to God-given standards. We didn't want to get caught up in the mindless ways of the world. We wanted our children to sense the overall importance of deeper things and to avoid the mistakes of our youth. We had such an enormous feeling of thanks to God for answering our prayers with yet another child.

The days I thought I'd never see were mine. Our home seemed to be bursting with activity and shrinking in size all at the same time. Through God's earlier provision of carpentry skills for Phil, adjustments were made and our home again accommodated our needs. With Rob in school, Elisabeth in preschool, and a new baby, life began to speed up. We thought Elisabeth would benefit from dance class and also enrolled her in swimming lessons. Another gift from Rob. Each of our children would learn to swim independently by the age of three and be strong swimmers by the age of five. These lifetime abilities came to them from a near tragedy.

~ ELEVEN ~

Rob's seizure medication began causing physical and emotional behavior problems. With the doctors, we made the decision to wean him off the prescription drug. He had one seizure after another with each decrease. We anxiously saw him through each episode. Finally he was completely off and the doctors were able to stabilize him with different medication. The process took almost a year but once it was over, even his drooling had improved though it had not stopped. We felt like we had rounded another corner in his life without going over the cliff.

Rob wove himself around each of the children as he had woven himself around us. In simple, unassuming ways we were linked without even being aware of it. We bought a piano for Elisabeth. Rob was delighted. Every day he would go to it and sit down and play his own tunes. On days when he was happy, he'd play soft light sounds, on days when he was frustrated or upset he'd play loud angry sounds. Music filled our home.

From the beginning, Elisabeth seemed to be inspired by music, too. I often wondered if Rob's love of it and her love of him had not made it so. It was their connection to each other and as it unfolded over the years, it became a force and passion that changed her life and shaped her into the person she is today. Each new day showed us that many great things would come from these small beginnings.

Bryan was a large boy from the start and walked at an early

age. His personality is gentle and loving. In a few short years, he began to take Rob's hand and carefully lead him wherever he needed to go. It touched all that saw them. They shared the same room for thirteen years. He never complained of Rob's humming at night. Preschool teachers who did not know our family makeup would speak of how exceptional Bryan was for his age. They would mention his kindness toward others and his maturity. Phil and I always knew that these were more of Rob's gifts flowing out into the world through Bryan. What kind of person would Bryan have become without Rob? How is each of us changed by the life of another?

With our minds on the children's activities, Phil's job, upkeep on the house, and church functions, we were very surprised by another pregnancy. Unlike previous ones, this one progressed with few problems, but I began to show at an early stage. Thinking that my body was just out of shape, we dismissed any other thoughts. My doctor suggested an ultrasound in the first trimester just as I had had with each of the other pregnancies.

I arrived for my appointment feeling somewhat nervous, as these tests always brought out a degree of anxiety. As the exam began, I could sense a change in the technician. I kept looking at the screen, and knew something was definitely different. She said very cautiously, "Has anyone said anything to you about twins?" Twins! How could I be having twins? There must be some mistake. But there they were. As she took all the measurements, the reality of what lay ahead began to flood over me.

Oh Lord, you must be laughing at us now, I thought. Be careful what you pray for, others had often said. Now I knew what they meant. I had always wanted children and now I would have them in abundance. Many concerns ran through my mind. Premature birth was more common with multiple pregnancies. Please Lord, keep them healthy and let them be at least seven pounds each, I prayed. Friends would laugh and say that five pounds was the most I could hope for.

We always put up the cradle in our sunroom about a month before each delivery. It was a prop to let Rob know that there would soon be a new arrival. By this time, Rob was catching on. But when we put up the cradle and a bassinet, he looked very confused. He walked back and forth between the two shaking his head in wonder. "Yes, Rob," I told him, "there are two this time."

We had never asked to know the sex of the babies, but through some of the technician's comments during a later ultrasound exam, I felt sure we must have been having a boy and a girl. Just in case we were wrong, we chose two boys' names but I was having trouble coming up with two girls' names. My due date was getting closer when one day, while talking to a friend, she mentioned the name Christine. Since the first baby we had lost was to be named Christina, I had not considered that name again. After our conversation I decided that in the remote possibility we had two girls, we'd use the name Christine.

On February 10, 1986, sixteen years after Rob's birth, we increased our family size from five to seven with the addition of two beautiful daughters. One we named Katherine Michelle and the other we named Christine Marie. Each weighed one ounce less than eight pounds! When I told my sister Barb what we had named them she almost cried. She later told me that she felt like God had given us back what had been taken away. We were more than doubly blessed with these new lives. We could hear God's laughter.

~ TWELVE ~

He settles the barren woman in her home as a happy mother of children. Praise the Lord.

PSALM 113:9

Without a doubt, we had outgrown our two-bedroom home. Our first home. The home where dreams had been shattered and then fulfilled. The home where we brought each of our children since Rob. The home we had tended and poured ourselves into for eleven years. The home we loved was now too small to hold us all.

When the twins were six months old, we moved to a home closer to our church and the church school they would all attend. Initially, we had loved the gift—our home—rather than the Giver. Now we gave credit where credit was due but leaving was still pain-filled. Within these walls we had made the journey of the prodigal son. It was hard to let go because we were so used to holding things tight. Harder lessons lay ahead.

Many members of our congregation pitched in and made the move easier. We had joined the church six years earlier and church members had always rallied around us in our times of need. We lived hundreds of miles away from our parents but that was the price we paid to stay in Michigan for its special education programs. The church was always there throughout our trials offering prayers, phone calls, cards, a hot dish, a helping hand. Now we again felt the arms of our congregation around us and we were reminded of God's faithfulness through His family. Their genuine concern for Rob also endeared them to us forever. They gave him warm handshakes, prayed for him during illness, and were concerned for his well-being.

We chose four women of great faith from this body to be Katherine and Christine's godmothers. One of them stopped by frequently to take Bryan for a walk or over to her house for a little visit so that I could do more packing. She taught him how to give butterfly kisses. So many people showed concern for us. But it was their love of the Lord that really struck us and motivated us to see what they saw and have what they had. We were like giant sponges, absorbing all we could, trying to make up for the time we wasted in our wandering years.

In letting go of an earthly home, I began more and more to think about my heavenly home. Our days were filled with activity but we continued to feel the pull of God's hand taking us to deeper levels with Him. Our hunger to study God's Word grew and we had a wealth of opportunities. I spent many Sundays, when the girls were babies, standing in the narthex of the church, holding one in each arm with Bryan clinging to my skirt so that I would not miss the sermon. Phil, Rob, and Elisabeth listened in church. I chose not to use the nursery that was provided because I believed the Spirit of God could work through His words into the hearts of my children. No matter what their age, His Spirit was working in them since the day of their baptism, the day when His grace and forgiveness had changed them forever.

But just getting to church was a challenge. To go anywhere meant at least three hours of preparation before departure.

But we saw the benefit of commitment and faithfulness and nothing except illness stopped us. Each Sunday we came, each Sunday we grew, and each Sunday we gave thanks not only for God's many physical blessings but also for the spiritual blessings we were beginning to see.

When vacation Bible school rolled around the summer after Katherine and Christine were born, Elisabeth and Bryan went. Bryan was almost three and the church made an exception to include him, if for no other reason than to give me time with fewer demands. When the children came home on Friday, they were excited by the rousing finale to the week. They told me that their lesson was all about heaven. Elisabeth took the lead and said how the lesson had made her think of Rob. She said, "We were talking about heaven and I said 'probably when we get to heaven we won't recognize Rob.'" Bryan became impatient and said "Uh, huh. We will. He will be changed and *we* will be changed."

I praise you, Father, Lord of heaven and earth, because you have hidden these things from the wise and learned, and revealed them to little children. Yes, Father, for this was your good pleasure.

MATTHEW 11:25-26

~ THIRTEEN ~

Rob's orthopedic development began to cause us concern. As he grew, we saw changes in muscle tightness in his legs as well as a beginning slope forward of his shoulders. Deformities were noticeable in every area of his body. The fact that he had ever learned to walk was more a testament to his will than to his construction. Still, our concerns led us to seek medical advice. We hoped to prevent any loss of mobility.

X-rays revealed that Rob was developing kyphosis—a slow, progressive rounding of the spine. He was evaluated at the University of Michigan and at the Minnesota Spine Center. Doctors told us that this condition would continue, resulting in paralysis. They advised us to consider a complex surgical procedure during which surgeons would remove a rib from Rob's front to increase flexibility. Then they would operate on his spine to stabilize it with a rod and to fuse several vertebrae. In our hearts, we didn't think that Rob would survive these operations. Without admitting it verbally, we both sensed that this might be the beginning of the end for Rob. After much thought and prayer, we decided to take one day at a time rather than risk surgeries that would cause Rob such suffering with no guarantee of success.

All our medical concerns for Rob led us to consider legal guardianship as Rob approached his eighteenth birthday. Many other parents we knew through the Association for Retarded Citizens had taken this step. They advised us to do so to protect our rights as his parents and to assure that the outside world could not take advantage of him. We gave the decision a lot of thought and concluded that, given the medical and legal climate of the country, we should indeed provide for Rob in this manner.

We met with social workers and social workers met with Rob to ask his opinion about having his mother and father make decisions for him. He answered all their questions in the affirmative and we were given a court date. We could only surmise that his answering the questions in such a manner had convinced them that he did indeed need our protection. Would an eighteen-year-old of sound mind say such a thing?

The three of us met in the courthouse before a judge and there we agreed to continue to provide for Rob's needs and to have legal responsibility for him as we had for the previous eighteen years. It was such a beautiful day that we decided we should tend to another task looming before us. Since Rob was now eighteen and was required by law, with no exceptions, to register for military service, we all walked over to the United States Post Office and registered him for the military draft. We realized both the magnitude and the absurdity of the day. The postmaster said he had seen worse apply.

By this point, we had settled into the suburban lifestyle and it felt wonderful. Phil's jobs in advertising had taken him from a television station, to a privately owned advertising agency, to a Christian publishing company. Rob was thriving at school despite regular absences due to illness. The school began to focus on getting the students out into the community more often. They took regular trips to department stores, to work outings at the Humane Society where they would wash animal bowls or walk and pet animals, to concerts, on picnics, to the zoo, and to restaurants. The goal was to expose the students to as many new experiences as possible in order to promote socially acceptable behavior in them.

Many of these children were now in their late teens and, depending on their size and ability, could be quite a handful. I remember one older mother confiding to me that she could no longer physically manage her son who now lived in a large man's body and would frequently sit down whenever he didn't want to walk any longer. Consequently, many parents, some of whom were considerably older than we, simply stopped trying to do these activities with their sons or daughters.

The secondary goal of such outings was to acclimate the community at large to the needs, appearance, and manner of our children. New laws now accommodated their participation in community events, but until they actually participated no one realized their needs. Schools led the effort through the work of devoted staff members. Without them, communities would never have known the numbers of people who would have missed out on these enjoyable, helpful activities. Without these exposures, a community could ignore or neglect the needs of these residents. And without such enlightenment and knowledge the communities would not become all that they should become.

Throughout Rob's years in school, we had been part of an evolutionary process regarding the treatment of people like our son. When Rob was born, many such children were immediately institutionalized. As mass institutionalization ended, schools specializing in care, education, and training began to emerge. Characteristically, these were isolated buildings, usually with many acres around them as a buffer for both sides. As laws ended discrimination against the handicapped, more classrooms began to open up in regular elementary and high school programs. These complied with the "least restrictive environment" aspect of the federal law. The idea was that as awareness increased, so would acceptance and opportunity.

By the time Rob was in his late teens, the local public high school created such a room. It provided educational opportunities for students in an isolated setting within that school. Nine to thirteen students would be transferred to the program with more to follow if the program was successful. Rob was one of the first to be chosen.

We had many concerns about such a move. Would he be placed in a situation where others could take advantage of him? Would he be made fun of or teased? Would he be physically abused? How would he be able to make a contribution? Again we saw that just his presence in the hallway, in the cafeteria, being loaded on to and off buses, would make a statement to others that this life was being lived despite all the obstacles, despite all the hardships. And it was being lived as fully as possible. Off he went to high school.

For years, Rob had loved to lock hands with any willing partner and dance to real or imagined music. But in high school, National Honor students came in to fulfill community service hours and Rob became a determined dancer. He started to notice girls and seemed to think that each was a candidate for the next dance. At home he would try to con Elisabeth or any of the rest of us into a musical interlude with him. Dancing became his passion. He would approach anyone coming to our home for a visit. He started to find partners at church. He was a young man on a mission who just couldn't stop those dancing feet. We never regretted our decision to let Rob be a part of this high school experiment. We only saw good come out of his participation.

We were always aware, however, of the need for discipline in Rob's life. Sometimes, parents of special needs children tend to ignore inappropriate behavior and concentrate only on the physical and mental development of their children. Many believe that bad or socially annoying behavior can't be changed. We believed that every child needed discipline, boundaries, and guidelines. We used physical discipline and verbal reprimands as we did with our other children.

For the most part, Rob learned to be well behaved but the need for constant reminders was part of our routine. When the mind of a two-year-old is in the body of a twenty-year-old, there's always room for concern. We were very aware of the fact that one bad experience with a handicapped person might renew fears or superstitions and deter others from interactions in the future. We hoped to lessen the negative feelings and heighten the positive ones through the examples of his life with us.

With Rob in high school, Elisabeth doing well in our church, operated school, and Bryan in preschool, our lives were busy but orderly. We were actively involved in our church and loved our neighborhood. We had redecorated every room in our new house by the time the twins were three. Everything seemed perfect and we rejoiced in all the blessings that now filled our lives. Life was so comfortable. We soon began to learn that mountaintop experiences do not last a lifetime.

~ FOURTEEN ~

Looking back over our lives, we can each think of events that signaled a change in direction. For us it began with Scraps, our cat of eleven years. One day she stopped eating. For a week, I tried to get her to eat but it was no use. Knowing what needed to be done, I took her to the vet who did the deed.

God had used Scraps to bring hope to us and change into our home all those years ago; now Scraps brought death and letting go into our home. God in His mercy softens all our sorrows through gradual steps that lead us to His arms. The Lord readied us for greater tests through the life of an animal that had come into our lives because she was abandoned, unwanted by her owner. God never wastes anything.

While Phil had continued to grow professionally through all the stages of his career, he began to feel less challenged. He wondered if the Lord might have other need of him, other ways to use his talents and abilities. After a business convention, a company that owned and operated Christian radio stations throughout the country approached him. After several discussions and a trip to California, they offered him the station manager position for their Chicago station.

Grand Rapids had been our home for nearly twenty years. We had put our roots down deep. Grand Rapids had programs that would last Rob's entire life. Special education would provide for his needs for four more years until the age of twenty-six, then Community Mental Health offered workshops and other opportunities. How could we think of leaving? Our other children were all in the church school by this time. Elisabeth was in seventh grade, Bryan in third, and Katherine and Christine in first. I was working in the school library. Did God really want us to leave all this?

Beyond the emotional concerns of leaving friends, church, school, and home, were the additional concerns for economic security. After years of relative comfort, were we placing ourselves in situations that would jeopardize all that we had worked so long to provide? Everything in me said, "I can't do this." Again I began to feel God's hand on me, reminding me that I needed to trust His plan, His way over my own.

One Sunday, at a crucial point in our decision-making process, it was Phil's turn at church to read the epistle lesson. In our congregation, elders rotated responsibility for these readings, and on this particular day, Phil was on duty. From the back of the church came the words from Hebrews. My knees still shake to this very day as I recall this reading, spoken as if only to me. I knew immediately in my heart what we must do.

> By faith Abraham, when called to go to a place he would later receive as his inheritance, obeyed and went, even though he did not know where he was going. By faith he made his home in the promised land like a stranger in a foreign country; he lived in tents, as did Isaac and Jacob, who were heirs with him of the same promise. For he was looking forward to the city with foundations, whose architect and builder is God....
>
> All these people were still living by faith when they

> died. They did not receive the things promised; they only saw them and welcomed them from a distance. And they admitted that they were aliens and strangers on earth. People who say such things show that they are looking for a country of their own. If they had been thinking of the country they had left, they would have had opportunity to return. Instead, they were longing for a better country—a heavenly one. Therefore God is not ashamed to be called their God, for he has prepared a city for them.
>
> HEBREWS 11:8-10, 13-16

God seemed to be reminding me that I was being too consumed by earthly dwellings and to be asking me for deeper commitments. How could I say no to God after all He had done for me?

A woman from our congregation gave us a wall hanging for our Chicago home as we tearfully left Grand Rapids. It said, "The light of God surrounds us, the love of God enfolds us, the power of God protects us, the presence of God watches over us. Wherever we are God is ... and all is well."

From the beginning, though, our transition was not an easy one. Our house sold in two weeks but the sale became complicated and fell through. Our house was back on the market over the holidays and we were separated for six months. Phil lived in Chicago, coming home to us in Grand Rapids on weekends. We had purchased a house in Chicago and now faced two house payments a month. Finally after months of trials, we were all reunited under one roof, apprehensive but hopeful.

~ FIFTEEN ~

When times are good, be happy; but when times are bad, consider: God has made the one as well as the other.

ECCLESIASTES 7:14

We chose our house after finding a congregation that also operated a school. Our connection to church, school, and home had been such a close one in Grand Rapids that we wouldn't start any other way. We hoped for the same closeness, the same harmony, the same strength and spirit. Once involved in the congregation, though, we saw that we would never share its goals and principles.

After three years of effort, during which we started several Bible study groups, the conflict within us was too great to remain. We felt let down and discouraged by the church. It lacked consistency in moving from teaching to doing, it lacked focus on Christ-centered activity, and it was unfaithful to God's call of evangelism. We said good-bye to their fundraising and their Halloween Haunted House and continue to pray for them to this day.

Grief over our losses held our hearts down, but we succeeded in finding a congregation more deeply committed to the preaching, teaching, and evangelism call of the gospel. Once again, we soaked up the words and felt the strength return.

The year before we left our first Chicago congregation, Phil shattered his ankle when he fell while trimming our trees. The doctors inserted a plate to promote growth and healing but Phil suffered numerous reactions to the antibiotics. Infection developed and continued until the doctors decided to remove the plate. Phil finally recovered after a year and a half of physical warfare. Every area of our lives seemed filled with struggle and hardship.

When we were feeling the most stress and sorrow over our church membership, my mom called to say that my father had lung cancer. He began treatment, but things did not look good for complete recovery. My mother's parents were also slipping away. On top of that, several of the on-air and sales staff at the station challenged Phil's authority. Conflicts over the direction and leadership of the station became daily battles.

I struggled with the constant constraints that came with having Rob home all day. Any outside activity for Rob had to be paid for out of the household income. That forced us to decide between a program for him and Christian education for the others. We reasoned that the others' needs were greater at the moment, even though this decision meant isolation for Rob and me. We were confronted on all sides by forces greater than anything we had ever known. We seemed to be sacrificing more than we were sure we could. "Why, Lord?" I asked, "When all we want to do is follow you?"

"Follow me?" I could almost hear Him say. "Then remember my words, 'any of you who does not give up everything he has cannot be my disciple'" (to paraphrase Luke 14:26). I was now with Rob in a closer way than I had ever been, with no outside intervention. I saw that this was a great gift of time to share with my son. God was using Rob to teach me lessons about contentment, patience, sacrifice, and love. As I tended his body and held him and fed him day after day, I began to feel Rob's peace despite all the trials of our life. He was unconcerned about the bills, or health issues, or jobs, or memberships. He lived in a body that defied the circumstances. He was content. God faithfully provided for him. He was a lily of the field. I began to want what he had, what I knew I lacked.

Still grieving over the loss of our beloved Grand Rapids and our church home, I received a call to come to my father's deathbed. We had visited more frequently since Dad's cancer was diagnosed, but we were so far away. His passing brought to the forefront the truth I knew in my heart, the victory that all believers share. The troubles of this world are many. We are determined to do things our way, we are alienated from God, we rely on self rather than Him. But that isn't enough to make Him stop loving us. He bends down to remind us of the price He paid to make us His own. "You are not your own; you were bought at a price. Therefore honor God with your body" (1 Cor 6:19-20).

Three short months after my father died, my grandfather died. One a man of faith, one a man unsure, but both powerful forces in my life, both leaving a great void. Their lives reminded me of the passage of time and the importance of living with purpose and meaning. Their deaths reminded me that we are only here a short time. Were we living our lives as we should? Were we the children of faith we ought to be? Did God's light shine through us?

~ SIXTEEN ~

But God chose the foolish things of the world to shame the wise; God chose the weak things of the world to shame the strong. He chose the lowly things of this world and the despised things—and the things that are not—to nullify the things that are, so that no one may boast before him.

1 Corinthians 1:27-29

The seizures, under control for years, returned. Illnesses became immediate threats, as Rob's temperature would soar with little warning. He began to have more trouble seeing and seemed uncertain of himself in unfamiliar settings. The back curvatures caused by scoliosis and kyphosis worsened with every passing year. He now had to strain to look up. By the end of a day spent watching TV, he looked weary. Still, he brought us a message of hope in the midst of trial through his enjoyment of life, his laughter over Grover's antics on Sesame Street and the Muppets, his determination to find the good.

Increasingly, he enjoyed watching two videotapes, one produced by Quigley Village called *Patiently Wait* and another about the miracles of Jesus. Rob repeatedly selected these videos when we asked him what he wanted to watch. In his own way, he was reminding me of the wisdom my mother had shared about hope and patience. I prayed for the miracles and tried to be patient.

Rob had always loved church. In Grand Rapids, he loved

using the kneeler during prayer time. He was never discouraged by the effort it took to position himself. He wanted to kneel. He wanted to pray. As the years passed and his attention span increased, he connected more with what was going on during worship. Always ready for music, he would quickly hand me a hymnal after we sat down for worship, nudging me gently with it if I remained too long in prayer. "Get ready to sing, Mom," he seemed to be saying.

One Easter morning, we attended the sunrise and the following service where Rob repeatedly heard the age-old refrain, "He is risen," followed by the congregation's response, "He is risen indeed." Rob shot to his feet in agreement. Whenever there was a baptism, he strained to watch. One such Sunday, he pointed to his chest as the baby was baptized. I felt that he, too, wanted to be included in this event. As a congregation, we said the words that reminded us of our connection to the Spirit at our baptism, but Rob couldn't say those words. It occurred to me that if I made the sign of the cross on his forehead and his heart at the same time the pastor was making it on the baby, Rob might get the connection too. He was delighted. From his reaction, I believe he understood.

He had always pointed to the front of the church during worship. Trying to teach him not to point was a continual process. In his later years I began to wonder what he was pointing at. I even wondered if he saw something that I could not. He was without language, but perhaps God gave him visions that only Rob could see—God's compensation. Of course, I would never know what he saw or thought or felt, I could only wonder.

And Rob remained faithful in prayer. He would not eat

until we prayed. He learned a sign prayer that began with us saying "Thank you," which Rob would sign by bringing his flat palm up to his mouth and then quickly bringing it down. We said "God" and Rob pointed heavenward. Next we said, "For food" and Rob pinched his fingers together and brought them up to his mouth, "and drink" for which he made a "c" shape with his hand to sign drink, "and sleep" and Rob crossed his hands and put his forehead on them. Finally we'd say "and Jesus." Rob would press his index finger very forcefully into his palms, first one then the other, giving the sign for Jesus. Then and only then would Rob open his mouth to eat.

One Sunday when Rob was unusually out of sorts and my patience had grown thin, an elderly woman walked over to us and said, "You remind me of my mother. My brother," she said, motioning to Rob, "was like him." Again I was struck with the way God weaves our lives together. I was thinking that the morning was somehow less than I had hoped it would be, but this woman reminded me that more was going on than I could ever realize. "It's not easy," she said, and walked away. Behind her knowing eyes, I saw the link that transcended space and time. I was now connected with this mother long gone. I realized that on some future day, my children might be so linked with some other mother in remembrance of me. These were gifts of memory, and love, and reminders of God's wisdom.

At times, I watched from a distance as one of Rob's siblings guided him through a crowd, into a car, to the bathroom, put their arms around him, wiped his chin, straightened his hair, talked tenderly to him. I knew these experiences were shaping them. I knew that God was using Rob in their lives, too, to give them understanding and maturity beyond their years.

~ SEVENTEEN ~

Therefore we do not lose heart. Though outwardly we are wasting away, yet inwardly we are being renewed.... For our light and momentary troubles are achieving for us an eternal glory that far outweighs them all. So we fix our eyes not on what is seen, but on what is unseen. For what is seen is temporary, but what is unseen is eternal.

2 CORINTHIANS 4:16-18

Phil's job ended. We knew it was coming. There was no way that all sides would ever agree on direction or mission. It was a relief in one area but it increased strain in another. Had we misinterpreted what God wanted us to do with our lives? Where should we go from here? Loss and letting go seemed to be all consuming. God remained faithful in our weakness, reminding us through Phil's day calendar of His promises. "See, I am doing a new thing! Now it springs up; do you not perceive it? I am making a way in the desert and streams in the wasteland" (Is 43:19).

Make it so, Lord, I prayed. It seemed to me that I had always been praying for the wrong things. I was still praying for my wishes, my will, not prepared to accept the will of the One who knew more than I.

But God knew our fears and needs and worked through our circumstances to bring us to a place of greater security. He sent a man willing to support Phil's effort to start a Christian advertising company. Building a company, we would learn, was to know total dependence on God's provision.

Most important, we again had health insurance through Phil's employment benefits. Health insurance was necessary with five children. Foremost on our minds were concerns for Rob's health and the unpredictability of his circumstances in the future. "Will they take Rob?" was always our first question whenever we discussed any employment or health policy changes. With a deep sigh, with renewed enthusiasm, and with many prayers of thanksgiving, we hoped for brighter days to come.

But that was not the plan, either. Rob's seizures came more frequently, often occurring in the car in the middle of rush-hour traffic. I would frantically look for a place to pull over so that I could position him to keep his airway clear. We had always been thankful that Rob was small in stature. Manhandling him at times like these was easier because of his size. I was now afraid to leave him even for short periods of time, even though his brother and sisters were very capable of caring for him. I was concerned that something serious or permanent might happen while he was in their care.

We were a busy household, though. Sports, music, church, school, and neighborhood filled our days and it became impossible to do it all without having them watch Rob. So I prayed as I ran here or there. "Don't let anything happen now, God, please don't let anything happen now." The doctors increased his medication but that made him sick to his stomach and caused him to gag with every meal. The seizures were not frequent enough to warrant the daily discomfort that the increase brought.

Because of living with Rob, I was more aware of details, I was an observer, I was watchful. He couldn't tell me how he felt, so it was my job to read the signs and know his need. Changes in his health kept me in a state of heightened readiness. We tried to eliminate the problems of the future with the watchfulness of today.

This meant regulating Rob's complete environment. Fluctuations of temperatures had always caused extreme fluctuations in Rob. He was hot or cold with no in-between. We used space heaters in the winter and fans in the summer. Air conditioning in our Chicago home eased much of his discomfort on the hottest summer days. As the years passed, we learned the hard way that his skin was developing acute sensitivity to the sun. If exposed to even moderate sunshine, he would blister and burn painfully. Rob's world seemed to narrow with every passing year. It was a challenge to provide shelter and protection for Rob and yet offer the opportunities for exploration and diversity that he and all our children needed.

The condition of readiness, this state of mind, spilled over into other areas of my life. The increased awareness, sensitivity, and preparedness for Rob caused an increased awareness throughout my own life. My observances of the intricacies of nature and the people around me and the world at large deepened and grew.

Paul's prayer became my prayer for myself and for my children: "that your love may abound more and more in knowledge and depth of insight, so that you may be able to discern what is best and may be pure and blameless until the day of Christ, filled with the fruit of righteousness that comes through Jesus Christ—to the glory and praise of God" (Phil 1:9-11).

Rob anchored us. As our lives became fuller, Rob's life, little by little, became more centralized, with all of us shooting out from him. When any of us came in, he was there watching public television or a Disney movie or a Quigley's Village or the Muppets. Our house was always full of the sound of this entertainment.

From the beginning, each of the children knew that the television was there for Rob's enjoyment. When they were little they, too, enjoyed many of the same things that he enjoyed. As they grew and matured, they were spared much of the entertainment that captured their friends. We always told them that they were perfectly capable of entertaining themselves while Rob was not. Without exception, they accepted these restrictions. To our surprise, they even continued to watch and enjoy many of the same things that Rob watched, if only to share some time with him.

He kept us innocent. He shielded all of us from the vulgarity and corruption that was taking over the airways. He helped us hold on to the purer truths. "Whatever is true, whatever is noble, whatever is right, whatever is pure, whatever is lovely, whatever is admirable ... think about such things" (Phil 4:8).

But our sea was shifting now. As Elisabeth departed to college, our thoughts became more future oriented. One of our children no longer slept in her bed in our home. The years seemed to be flying by and soon our children would all be on their own. All except for Rob. Over the years, Phil and I had joked about our life. Like other couples, we talked about what the years ahead would be like. We mused about our retirement saying, "You, me, and Rob." Our lives together seemed inseparable, linked forever. As the other children had reached their teens, we had allowed ourselves occasional evenings out to enjoy a church gathering or school function. We cherished these moments because we had waited for them for so long.

But from time to time, I wondered about the years to come. Should we find a care center for Rob after the other children were grown? Should we think about having a life separate from his someday? Among the many things that we were thankful for was the fact that we were so young when Rob was born. Our youth, with its strength and endurance, got us through many difficult years. But after nearly thirty years, we began to wonder about the next twenty.

I had seen many older parents struggle with their inability to physically care for their handicapped children. Would we too find ourselves in this situation? What was best for Rob? How long would we be able to think only of his needs? There were endless questions but no easy answers.

~ EIGHTEEN ~

You are a mist that appears for a little while and then vanishes.

JAMES 4:14

As Rob approached his thirtieth year, he seemed more interested in hugs and dancing, content to be outside the mainstream. In fact, contentment covered him like a blanket and as I fed him, I shared in it too. The questions and trappings of the world were meaningless. Power, beauty, intellect, wealth, would all fade away in time. All the things that I would have run after before Rob's life were now revealed as shallow and empty. We had lived long enough to see the sham of such pursuits and to know that the only treasure of worth was God's gift of salvation and love. In the end, we would all be stripped of our self-importance. In the end, we would all give account for what we'd done with what we'd been given.

Rob possessed great gifts of peace and righteousness. He had never struck out at another person; any anger he showed he directed at himself. He never lied, or cheated, he never boasted, he never cursed or used questionable language. Rob never coveted, gossiped, or stole. He never gave anything but love. Isaiah wrote "the fruit of righteousness will be peace; the effect of righteousness will be quietness and confidence forever" (Is 32:17).

Rob was evidence of these truths.

Days with Rob brought me more peace than I'd ever known

before. Rob had always loved to look through the photo albums and could always find a picture of himself. One day, we traveled back through the years and I was struck by all the memories that came. Phil had changed from a boy who wasn't sure he wanted children to a man who doted on five of them. He would do anything for them and was quick to boast of their accomplishments. He was always ready to be what the situation required. He would crawl into a box with Rob and make sound effects to make him laugh. He built sandboxes and swing sets at each of our homes. He changed diapers, cleaned up messes, made Saturday morning pancakes, and prayed daily for each of his children.

He was gentle and loving with Rob. Rob had made him a father and the role suited him and matured him. We each might have tried to take credit for our children without Rob as a reminder. Rob made us thankful for the gift of life—his, ours, and our other children's—but more important, he reminded us that as parents we were simply the vessels through which God's handiwork flowed. They were His creation, not ours. Important, too, was the fact that we are all here on loan, a temporary stopping spot before our journey home.

God stood before us one beautiful, sunny, Sunday morning in September. We all prepared for church in our routine way. Rob ate his regular bowl of oatmeal and smashed banana, followed by a carton of yogurt and his meds. He seemed eager as always to go to church. We took separate cars because I had a Sunday school teachers meeting after the worship service. Bryan, who had a learner's permit, drove in the lead car with Phil and Rob, and I followed behind with Katherine and Christine.

Before reaching downtown, I noticed that something was wrong with Rob who was sitting in the middle seat in the mini-van. Phil and Bryan, realizing it, too, pulled over. I knew it was another seizure. I pulled up behind them and went to help. Phil and I moved to opposite sides of the van, turning Rob in the seat, following all the routines we'd come to know so well. But this seizure did not follow the same patterns and we became concerned. The seizure had stopped but Rob's breathing hadn't returned to normal. We both agreed that we should get him to the hospital.

Phil, Bryan, and Rob went to the hospital and I took the girls to church. Rob had been through so many emergencies, I had begun to think he would always pull through. Midway through teaching my Sunday school class, a neighbor came to my classroom door saying that I should get to the hospital immediately. Phil had been unable to get through the church's answering machine and had called her to get the message to me. Knowing that something must be terribly wrong, I headed for the hospital after finding someone to take my class.

"What's happened?" I kept thinking as I drove to the hospital. "God please keep him safe," I prayed. "Is he alive?" "Why didn't I stay with him?" "Lord have mercy, Lord have mercy." The sunshine surrounding me gave me no warmth.

When I entered the hospital and gave the receptionist my name, a nurse escorted me down a hallway to a room where Bryan and Phil were waiting. The nurse put her hand on my shoulder. "Oh, no," I remember thinking, "something is very wrong."

Phil stood and hugged me when I walked in. A look of

horror and shock was on Bryan's face. Without words, I knew that the Rob we had known was gone forever. It instantly occurred to me that as we had been making our way to our earthly sanctuary, he had been making his way to his heavenly one.

But Phil's words brought me back to reality. Rob was not physically dead. Because he had not been breathing and since CPR was virtually impossible because of his kyphosis, his heart had stopped beating by the time he reached the hospital. Doctors had worked on him for over twenty minutes until finally his heart started to beat again. He was put on a ventilator and taken to the ICU.

The doctors gave the bleakest of all possible reports. Twenty minutes, at least, without oxygen left little hope for any return to life as we had known it. We were asked about our wishes for future intervention. I wanted to scream at them for doing all this to my precious son. I felt sick. Why hadn't they let him die peacefully? Why, why, why? Phil and I agreed on a Do Not Resuscitate order.

As there had been reasons for Rob's life, so there were also reasons in its close. I knew this fact instinctively by now but the questions came anyway. Phil went to pick up Katherine and Christine at church and to ask our pastors for prayer. We made lists of who we needed to tell and arrangements we needed to make. Whether Rob lived in his present condition or died, nothing would ever be the same. I knew I would never see his earthly smile again. We had many things to think about and pray about.

My foremost thoughts were for my children and how this would affect them. They were so young to be confronted with such a great event. Would it draw them closer to their Savior or would they push Him away? We called Elisabeth. We knew that being so far away would be hardest for her now. When we told her about Rob's condition, she recalled that just the day before, on a choir retreat, she had been around a bonfire discussing the meaning of music in her life. That was now her chosen course of study in college. She told us that one of the other choir members mentioned that he had worked with handicapped children in a camp over the summer. Until then, he had always taken his musical ability for granted. One of the campers had loved hearing him sing and had said that they would someday sing together in heaven. Elisabeth had been touched by these words as her thoughts drifted back to Rob.

She had always been aware of her gift for music, whether playing or singing, and she knew that others were denied the abilities and privileges she possessed. As she spoke of her experience, we realized God was already preparing her for Rob's departure through the "story of heaven" spoken through a choir member about a person she had never met.

She often thought of Rob singing in full voice with the angels, as he had never been able to do with us here. She looked forward to the day when they would sing together in heaven to the praise and glory of their Lord. Maybe it had begun all those years ago with the vacation Bible school story of heaven, maybe even before that.

Over the years, she had written numerous papers about her brother's life and its meaning for her. When required to write several essays for entrance into the National Honor Society, she wrote one on Rob. It seemed both ironic and fitting that membership in a group noted for academic, civic, and personal excellence would be partially based on an essay written about her brother's life. He could never be admitted to such a group, but because of him and his influence in her life, because of the way her life had been shaped and changed by his, she could. Everything had come full circle.

Our parents and sisters needed to be notified. I wanted to call my mother, but she had just left on a nine-day trip to Washington, D.C. I was concerned about how and when to contact her. She had never traveled and this was her first real adventure since Dad died. I knew that she would be upset at not being with me in my hour of need, but I didn't want to ruin her getaway with news that would keep. I would contact her if ... or when....

What we needed most was prayer. Both our present congregation and our congregation in Grand Rapids joined us with fervent, earnest intervention. Prayers for wisdom in decision making were critical: what should be done for Rob and when? The power of prayer uplifted and strengthened us through the hours and days that followed. Our pastors came daily and shared devotions.

I felt detached from Rob when I first saw him lying in the hospital bed with his eyes closed. There was a tube in his mouth and down his throat. It was attached to a machine making a rhythmic, mechanical sound, moving his chest up and down. It all seemed too cruel. I believed that what I saw before me was no longer my son, only the remains of the container that once held him. No more personality, no more smile, no more Rob. He looked peaceful, as if the worst were over for him. On that first day, I could only stand at a distance or sit quietly in the room and read my Bible. I was confident of

Rob's eternal rest and escaped to the idea that he was already in the presence of his Maker.

But that was wishful thinking on my part. His body was operating because it had been forced back to its labor. His temperature soared, he convulsed, he began retaining the fluids that he was receiving intravenously. His tongue began to swell and envelop the invasive tube. He hiccupped. Only God knew where his spirit was. But this body that had grown inside me, that had fulfilled my dream of motherhood, this body that had been tended and held by me for nearly thirty years, now struggled somewhere between life and death.

The shock of the past two days was wearing off and I drew closer to him. I began to touch him, to kiss him. It became clear to me what a gift these moments were. I would miss this in the future, I would long for one more chance to brush his hair, to kiss his cheek, to hold his hand, so I would do it today while I still had the blessing. Thank you, God, for this most holy day.

There were some cards, some telephone calls, some visits to the hospital by those closest to us who were filled with sympathy. All offered us opportunities to share our faith and to feel the love of God extended through the love of others. But there was no gigantic outpouring; everyone, it seemed, was in shock, waiting. Again we had to lead the way, to show others how to approach us. We had opportunities to witness of our confidence and our hope and we were renewed daily.

~ NINETEEN ~

Strengthen the feeble hands, steady the knees that give way; say to those with fearful hearts, "Be strong, do not fear; your God will come ... he will come to save you."

ISAIAH 35:3-4

I could not sleep more than a couple of hours at a time, though. I would wake with Scripture verses or hymns going through my head and I knew that we should be preparing Rob's funeral service. I felt driven by a power outside my own. Over the years we had made mental notes of favorites for each of us if ever the time came to plan a service. Still, when the time arrives, the finality of it, the absoluteness of it, one thinks and rethinks the choices.

This most solemn and meaningful day should be one of profound thought, not done lightly, because this would be the last time his life would be publicly regarded. People would stop what they were doing and come to hear what we had to say about this life. It was important that we not waste the opportunity. But the most important thoughts were not ones about Rob, they were ones about the One who had claimed him all those years ago, the One who had protected and guided him, the One in whose arms Rob would eventually rest.

Day after day, through person after person, news of Rob spread and lives were touched through the church, schools, workplace, and neighborhood. We again felt a purpose for his life even now, as he lay in a bed with less ability than he had ever had. There was power and meaning for each mother I knew who held her child a little closer, grateful for the gift of another day. As Rob lingered, nurses and doctors saw our love and heard our stories about the meaning of his life; I believe that this will influence their thoughts about other such lives. We could still see the ripples flowing out of his life, as he lay lifeless on that bed.

All Rob's reflexes were gone, his pupil was blown, and there was only minimal brain stem activity. He had taken an occasional breath on his own while on the ventilator but the doctors believed that he would not be able to sustain breathing on his own. We had to decide whether to keep him on the ventilator until the rest of his body shut down, which was inevitable, or to take him off the ventilator. The reality was that we would soon need either a nursing home or a funeral home. Time had given us the ability to be mentally ready for either one.

On Thursday, we went to the hospital with the resolve and peace to make the decision. Significant time had passed and the physicians—cardiac, neurology, pulmonary, internal—all agreed. They set into motion the process of paperwork and details.

Left alone with Rob, I was again struck by the closeness I felt to God and Jesus, His Son. This relationship that we have with our children is such a close one, how do we give it up? *God must have felt the same way about Jesus,* I thought. He was pleased with His Son. We, too, were pleased with our son though we had to learn to be. His Son had suffered injustice and cruelty. So had ours. I knew that God knew my pain. I knew He cared, because He surely must have suffered as He watched His Son pay for my sins. Both what Jesus had done and what Rob was going through drew me back to God's loving embrace.

I cried, deep sobs, and I whispered to Rob that I loved him and that he had been such a good son. And with that, he let out a deep sigh that equaled my sobs. *OK, Rob, I will let you go now,* I thought. I can do no more. My love can't hold you any longer, my will to keep you is selfish and wrong. I will always carry you in my heart.

Our pastor walked in and Phil returned from the phone calls he had been making. We prayed a devotion based on Psalm 136 and read the words:

> Give thanks to the Lord, for he is good.
> *His love endures forever.*
> Give thanks to the God of gods.
> *His love endures forever.*
> Give thanks to the Lord of lords:
> *His love endures forever.*
> to him who alone does great wonders,
> *His love endures forever.*
> who by his understanding made the heavens,
> *His love endures forever.*
> who spread out the earth upon the waters,
> *His love endures forever.*
> who made the great lights—
> *His love endures forever.*
> the sun to govern the day,
> *His love endures forever.*
> the moon and stars to govern the night....

On and on in my heart went the stories of Scripture that I now knew so well, from Creation, to Passover, to David. These were God's promises to His chosen people, faithfully fulfilled through His love in Jesus. We could not doubt God's guiding hand or the promises He extended to Rob through his baptism. "Let the little children come to me, and do not hinder them, for the kingdom of heaven belongs to such as these" (Mt 19:14), Jesus said and we believed.

The intensive care nursing staff had made their rotation and a different nurse came in to see Rob through his day. She was tender and caring, as the others had been, but she spoke more directly to me. We soon realized that we had much in common. Our Elisabeth and her son had been in school together and she had enjoyed hearing Elisabeth's solos in high school concerts. We were fellow Lutherans on top of that. She assured us that she would keep Rob as comfortable as he could possibly be and she had a way about her that gave me peace when he was in her care. She was sure of herself and she understood our faith, our fears, and our heartache.

Preparations were now underway to remove the ventilator tube and she assisted the doctors with the necessary paperwork and readiness. We were asked to leave the room while the tube was removed. As we stood again at his bedside, this tenderhearted nurse pulled out a pocket Bible and asked us if she could read the Twenty-third Psalm.

Once off the ventilator, Rob's breathing slowed and weakened quickly and within five minutes his heart stopped for the final time. We prayed the Our Father and when the nurse left the room to give us some time alone, Phil began the words of the major doxology: "Praise God from whom all blessings flow,

Praise God all creatures here below, Praise God above ye heavenly hosts, Praise Father, Son, and Holy Ghost." I wanted to sing out in full voice but the words got caught in my throat. My heart filled with their meaning and my soul sang.

The journey that seemed so long had now ended too quickly. Thirty years compared with eternity is but a blink of the eye. The life that defied the predictions now rose in victory. "Then will the eyes of the blind be opened and the ears of the deaf unstopped. Then will the lame leap like a deer, and the mute tongue shout for joy.... They will enter Zion with singing; everlasting joy will crown their heads. Gladness and joy will overtake them, and sorrow and sighing will flee away" (Is 35: 5-6, 10).

~ TWENTY ~

One final time I chose clothing for Rob to wear. He had always worn turtlenecks and sweaters to guard against the cold so it only seemed right to clothe him thus. We ordered flowers, requesting that Fuji mums be spread throughout the arrangements. The visitation and the funeral would be held at church, because it was Rob's second earthly home. My sisters' husbands, their three sons, and Bryan would be pallbearers, now having performed this service three times in the past five years.

We would bury him in a well-established, evergreen-lined cemetery of rolling hills that lay across the street from our church. It was a town where none of our other relatives were buried, a town in which our future was uncertain. But we were learning to take care of our todays. Today we were here and this is where Rob had died. Like the pioneer fathers of our country and our faith, we would commit him to the ground which was the Lord's no matter if we remained there to tend the soil or whether we were called to some other mountain or valley.

We would sing songs of praise for Rob's life. "Rejoice, O Pilgrim Throng," "Glorious Things of Thee Are Spoken," "I Know that My Redeemer Lives," and "For All the Saints" were our choices though we could have easily chosen more. We planned a celebration of joy for what Rob now experienced. When we called Elisabeth and informed her of her brother's passing, she said, "Pick a hymn for me to sing. I want to sing."

I had finally reached my mother by phone. We would hold off on the service for Rob until she could be with us. She was filled with sorrow at not being with us in the hospital. Memories flooded over her and renewed her original grief when he was born and she was kept outside the hospital, not allowed the physical contact that would have given us both so much comfort. Why, she wondered, had she been kept from her daughter in such great times of need? What was the purpose?

As she struggled with these thoughts and prepared to make her way to our side, she and my youngest sister, Trish, arranged a flower display that conveyed the heart of her feelings. She used the bowl that had contained the Spirit-filled water for her own infant baptism sixty-nine years earlier. In it, they placed ten yellow roses, one for each of her living earthly grandchildren. In the center of the ten yellow roses, nestled with baby's breath, was one white rose for her heavenly grandchild, Rob.

We were joined by faith, this woman and I. As we met and embraced, I reminded her that she was always with me, because she was so much a part of my thoughts and actions. It occurred to me that God had kept us physically separate at these emotionally need-filled times so that I would rely on Him as my anchor rather than on her. She would always be an example to me, of strength, courage, determination, and faith.

The days of preparation between Rob's death and his funeral were days of reflection and comfort. We went through the photo albums that Rob had always loved and pulled out our favorite memories of him to display at his funeral luncheon. Picture after picture reminded us of the fullness and the meaning of his life.

Cards filled our mailbox daily. Hundreds of people opened their hearts as they shared their sorrow at Rob's passing. We were most touched by the responses of people that we had never even realized that Rob had affected. Those who said they felt such a sense of loss over his passing. Those who said they would miss seeing us together on a Sunday morning.

Some letters reminded us of the power of Rob's life.

"Seeing your family at the reunion was a very moving experience for me," wrote my cousin. "Love just seemed to radiate from within your family. Both you and Phil possess a gift that few people can ever attain. Your love and understanding of Robbie passes on to your other children and they too possess the gift.... Your family has shown me the true meaning of 'right to life.'"

"I heard about Robbie's passing this year and my prayers go out to you. I have so many memories of you and your family—mostly how much you loved and cared for your son," wrote one of Rob's former teachers. "He was one of my first students that meant so much to me and through the years I've had many, but Robbie stood out. I think a lot of it is because of how your family wove itself around him."

"He had an amazing life, living and giving way beyond anyone's expectations!" wrote our longtime friend Jan. "Your life was forever changed when Rob was born, and again when he died. It's what you did with the in-between time that has always led me to respect and marvel at you two; your patience, understanding, and ability to make life beautiful even through the difficulties."

From Grand Rapids, a sister in the faith wrote: "There are pictures printed indelibly on my mind of Rob and your love and care for him—the tilt of his head, his raised hand, your guiding arms, and the folded handkerchief you used to wipe his chin. At the time you were with us at Our Savior, your examples of caring spoke much to me. But I didn't really appreciate all you did until now when I find myself doing some of the same things in caring for my husband with Alzheimer's disease. I also was not aware of the unexpected rewards of joy and loving-kindness that God gives in place of our plans."

Whether by phone, in person, or in writing, expression after expression conveyed the same emotions and perceptions. All who took the time to look, who opened their eyes wide enough to let in the light, saw meaning for Rob's life. It was again a call to me to open my eyes wider and let more light in. The elderly, the sick, the stressed, the handicapped are all around us. Do I really see them? Do I really value the examples of their journey?

Rob had died on a Thursday and as is the case whenever there is a death of a loved one, we felt the surreal events of the world around us as activities once meaningful now seemed empty. Everything went on despite our great loss.

Bryan was scheduled to play in a football game on the following Friday night. He had been very private with the events of the week and had not shared them openly with his friends, teachers, or coaches. Feeling that the emotional drain had also affected his physical strength, he decided to talk to the coach before the game to give advance warning of possible shortcomings during the game. The coach acknowledged Bryan's loss. In his talk to the team before the game the coach announced to them that one of their members was hurting after the death of his brother and that they would dedicate the game to Rob's memory.

The game began. Bryan played with more strength than he thought he was capable of, making several good plays. His team won. Afterwards, the coach came over to him and presented him with the game ball. Bryan turned to Phil, who had come to support him, and said, "Here, Dad, this is in memory of Rob." After a tearful thank-you to the coach, they came home to share their experience with me. Again Rob's life, or memory of it, had been a spark.

Phil wrote the obituary notices to be included in four communities. When first reading Rob's, after it appeared, we noticed another beside his. It was that of a two-month-old child whose grandparents were members of our congregation. This infant had been on our prayer chain throughout the past few months but with all the events of the last week, I had not learned of her passing. I was struck with an overwhelming feeling of thankfulness as I again realized the gift the years had been for us. Rob could have just as quietly slipped out of our lives in his first few months as well. I could only imagine how our lives would have been changed.

As we prepared to leave for the visitation, the phone rang. It was a reporter from the local paper, assigned to write a story on Rob! He asked for a picture to include with the article, asking also for someone else to interview for more insight into Rob's life. The piece would appear in the next day's paper. Phil and I just laughed and wondered why we were surprised by such a happening. Rob had always attracted attention.

Hundreds of people came for Rob's visitation. We realized that hundreds more were kept away by the distance between us, especially those in Grand Rapids. Those who took time out of their busy lives to share their sympathy overwhelmed and strengthened us. Bryan's football coaches, teachers, our children's friends and parents, neighbors, members of our congregation, relatives who'd come hundreds of miles all reached out to us in love and compassion. When my sister's husband, Dave, came he was carrying a bouquet of Fuji mums. He, too, remembered that day so long ago when Rob had made this choice out of all the possible choices.

On the Tuesday morning of his funeral, car after car filled the church parking lot carrying Michigan license plates. These joined all the others from so many areas of our lives. Now we all united our voices as we sang our thanks for the life now silenced.

Elisabeth's voice rose from the church's balcony after the opening responses, as she sang "Lord of the Dance." With each verse we were drawn to the focus of our worship, with each verse we were reminded of the dance we were all part of, the dance Rob had been part of as he encouraged us to dance with him. "'They cut me down and I leapt up high; I am the life that will never, never die, And I'll live in you if you live in Me, for I am the Lord of the dance,' said He. 'Dance, dance, wherever you may be; I am the Lord of the dance,' said He. 'And I'll lead you all wherever you may be, And I'll lead you all in the dance, said He." Even so, Lord, lead us now.

Our pastor's words focused on Rob's baptism, the New Testament promise connection. Jesus had done it all for us. As Rob had received the gift of physical life, so also had he received the gift of spiritual life. We trusted God's mercy but more than that, we had all the assurances from recorded

Scripture that God is faithful to His promises.

Through baptism, He had promised Rob eternal life. The gift of grace was just that, a gift. In baptism, Rob received a gift that he, like we, had no ability to receive without the intervention of the Holy Spirit. We had seen evidence of the work of that Spirit in Rob's life and we knew with confidence whose arms now held him. "The one the Lord loves rests between his shoulders" (Dt 33:12). Where would we have found comfort without these promises or this faithfulness?

At the close of our worship our relatives, now turned pallbearers, once more carried the casket holding Rob's body to the hearse for the short ride to the cemetery. Predictions of rain and cold all proved false and on this warm, sunny, autumn day we closed another chapter of Rob's life. Now all that would remain for us would be the slow rebuilding of our lives, as we became accustomed to the emptiness of our home without his presence.

There would be more ease and more freedom for us, but we were forever changed by the life now stilled. I began to feel older for the first time in my life. Rob had made me feel that time stood still. Suddenly I realized that all my children, all these lives that I thought I'd never know, were nearly grown. In a few short years they would all be leaving home. I was more uncertain than I had ever been in regard to worldly affairs, but more certain than ever of spiritual ones. Rob was the instrument that God had used to get my attention.

~ TWENTY-ONE ~

As the end of the church year approached, I remembered our church's tradition of reading aloud the list of all the faithful who had passed from this kingdom to the next in the last year. Rob's name would be read and a bell would toll. It was always a moving service and now my son's name would be included. His name was chosen for the connection it brought between the generations of our family. Both maternal and paternal fathers, two uncles, Phil's middle name and mine were remembered in his.

"A good name is more desirable than great riches; to be esteemed is better than silver or gold" (Prv 22:1). We had named him thinking of the men whose lives had influenced ours. We had named him hoping that he would carry the best of them inside of him. Now we looked farther and we saw how he connected us to the only One that really mattered.

But I again marveled at how God had prepared me for Rob's death through the experiences of those I loved and admired. While I was in high school, my godfather and uncle—one of the uncles Rob was named after—died from heart complications in his late forties. He had been my grandmother's firstborn son and had had eating difficulties at birth. After his initial struggles, he grew to be a gentle, well-respected man. He held positions of importance both in the military and in the community but had never been puffed up by them.

My grandmother loved him deeply. My father thought he

was her favorite though no one seemed to mind because he was everyone's favorite. He was a quiet man and his smile lit up his face, too. Without words, he always made me feel loved. It was in the way he looked at me, the feeling I had when he stood beside me. When he died, I was crushed. But my grandmother told story after story about him and there was such peace and joy in her telling. I never saw her cry over him. Now I thought about those days. Now I understood. It seemed to me that more than anyone I'd ever known, she'd experienced the loss of all those she loved most. And she had survived. I knew, too, that part of her lived in me.

We journeyed through our first Thanksgiving and Christmas without Rob. In February, Rob's birthday came and went and we looked forward to spring and Easter, now learning what each season would be without him. One of our friends who had been a foster mother of two handicapped adults, who also died young, gave us many daffodils to plant in Rob's memory. We positioned them close to a smaller patch that had been planted years before we bought the house.

Extraordinarily warm temperatures led to an early spring. By the beginning of April, the older bulbs were inches taller than Rob's bulbs and we laughed to see the slowness of Rob's. How fitting, we joked. Then, as his were ready to bloom, they were hit with a snowstorm and we feared that they would be lost. The next day, in the afternoon sunshine, we were touched by the sight of the flowers. Now in full bloom, but with heads drooped, they reminded us of the configuration of Rob's frame and we had to smile. Reminders, again, that God uses the smallest details of our lives to bring us comfort and peace. Rob helped us to see the significance in all the insignificant.

Days later, as I held my Bible in my hands, I read the words from Isaiah:

> He has sent me to bind up the brokenhearted, to proclaim freedom for the captives and release from darkness for the prisoners, to proclaim the year of the Lord's favor ... to comfort all who mourn, and provide for those who grieve in Zion—to bestow on them a crown of beauty instead of ashes, the oil of gladness instead of mourning, and a garment of praise instead of a spirit of despair. They will be called oaks of righteousness, a planting of the Lord for the display of his splendor.
>
> ISAIAH 61:1-3

Rob had always been a reminder to us of how thankful we should be to have our voices, our mobility, our intelligence, our abilities. But he was also a reminder of how far we were from his innocence, his selflessness, his purity, his patience, and his love. His imperfections were far fewer than mine. In many ways, he reflected Christ's humility and unconditional love not through words or actions but just by being the person God created him to be.

But only through God the Father's gift, only through Jesus' love and sacrifice, only through the Spirit's power could Rob, or we, be called "a planting of the Lord." We knew with certainty that this is what he was, for through him we witnessed the Lord's splendor each day throughout his life.

All praise and glory be to the Father, Son, and Holy Spirit, one God forever.